NoMAD

From Thinning to Thriving: The Definitive
Guide to Hair Restoration, Nutrition, and
Advanced Therapies

NoMAD

From Thinning to Thriving: The Definitive Guide to Hair
Restoration, Nutrition, and Advanced Therapies

Copyright © *Levitas One*, 2024
All Rights Reserved

What are the NoMAD Plans?

Developed by Dr Ash Kapoor, the NoMAD Plans represent a transformative approach to health and wellness that combines the wisdom of ancestral practices with contemporary medical insights. The name "NoMAD" not only suggests a journey through the intricate realm of health but also stands for its foundational principles: Nutritional Optimisation, Mindful Adaptation, and Detoxification.

At the heart of NoMAD is the 6R Framework—Restore, Release, Repair, Renew, Reframe, and Represent.. This methodology addresses the root causes of illness, combats chronic inflammation, and cultivates authentic vitality, guiding individuals through a transformative process.

Tailored specifically to each individual, NoMAD journeys are meticulously crafted to rebalance the body, strengthen the mind, and rejuvenate overall health. By integrating ancestral practices with cutting-edge, innovative treatments—all under strict medical oversight—NoMAD Plans offer a personalised pathway to sustainable, long-lasting well-being that resonates with your unique life circumstances.

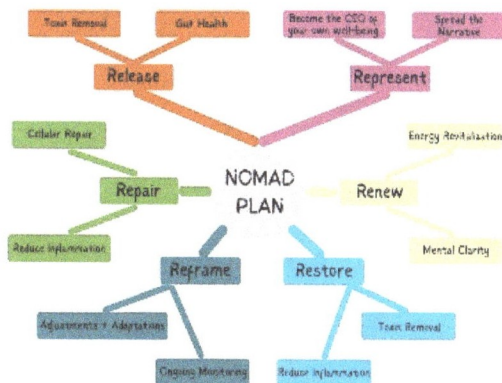

Levitas One:
"As Is In, As Is Out"

Reflecting the belief that our internal well-being is mirrored in our external environment. Founded by Dr. Ash Kapoor, Levitas One serves as the vehicle for delivering NoMAD's treatment plans. It envisions a healthcare future where patients are at the centre of a fully integrated, multidisciplinary approach. Guided by Nomads 6 Rs—Restore, Release, Repair, Renew, Reframe, and Represent—Levitas One empowers self-care through personalised guidance and minimal intervention, promoting long-term health, balance, and sustainability.

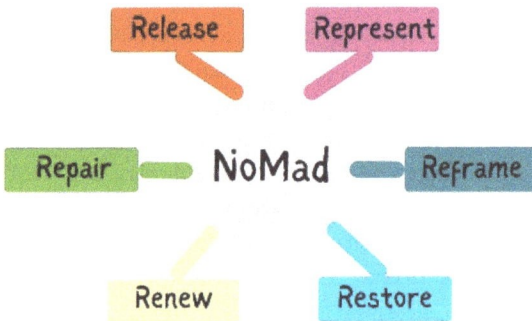

Contents

Introduction

Embracing a New Approach to Hair Restoration

Hair is often seen as more than just an aesthetic feature; it is a symbol of youth, health, and vitality. When hair begins to thin or fall out, it is not just a physical loss—it is an emotional one. For many, hair loss is a distressing experience that impacts confidence and self-esteem. Unfortunately, traditional pharmacological treatments often fail to provide satisfactory results because they focus on managing symptoms rather than addressing the root causes.

This book, *From Thinning to Thriving: The Definitive Guide to Hair Restoration, Nutrition, and Advanced Therapies*, offers a groundbreaking and holistic approach to understanding and managing hair health. It integrates cutting-edge science, nutrition, and ancestral wisdom to provide a comprehensive guide for anyone struggling with hair loss or looking to optimise hair growth. Our goal is to empower you with the knowledge and tools to not only halt hair thinning but also to restore your hair to its fullest, healthiest state.

The Philosophy of Hair Health: More Than Just Looks

Healthy hair is a direct reflection of overall health. Just as the health of a tree's leaves can indicate the state of its roots and soil, the quality of our hair reflects the state of our internal environment. When hair is strong, vibrant, and abundant, it often suggests that the body is well-nourished and balanced. Conversely, when hair becomes thin, brittle, or starts to shed excessively, it can signal systemic issues, such as hormonal imbalances, nutrient deficiencies, chronic inflammation, or underlying health conditions.

This book emphasises the importance of viewing hair as a marker of overall wellness rather than an isolated concern. Hair health is influenced by numerous factors, including:

1. **Nutritional Status**: Deficiencies in essential nutrients such as iron, biotin, vitamin D, and omega-3 fatty acids can significantly impair hair growth.

2. **Hormonal Balance**: Hormones like dihydrotestosterone (DHT), thyroid hormones, and oestrogen play critical roles in regulating the hair growth cycle.

3. **Scalp Health**: A healthy scalp provides the foundation for strong hair growth. Issues such as dandruff, seborrheic dermatitis, and poor circulation can disrupt follicular function and contribute to hair thinning.

4. **Stress and Lifestyle**: Chronic stress and unhealthy lifestyle habits can elevate cortisol levels, triggering conditions like telogen effluvium, where hair prematurely enters the resting phase.

Why Traditional Pharmacological Approaches Often Fall Short

Conventional hair loss treatments like Minoxidil and Finasteride are widely prescribed, but they often yield mixed results. Minoxidil works by increasing blood flow to the scalp, while Finasteride reduces the conversion of testosterone to DHT—a hormone that causes follicular miniaturisation in androgenetic alopecia. While these medications can slow hair loss and, in some cases, promote regrowth, they do not address the multifactorial nature of hair loss, nor do they improve overall scalp and hair health.

Furthermore, these medications can have undesirable side effects. Minoxidil may cause scalp irritation and dryness, while Finasteride is associated with potential sexual dysfunction and mood changes. For those who experience these side effects, discontinuing the treatment often leads to rapid hair loss, indicating that the solution was only temporary and did not address the root cause.

The Promise of Modern Science: High-Innovation Therapies for Hair Regeneration

Recent advancements in regenerative medicine and aesthetics have opened new doors for effective hair restoration. Therapies such as Platelet-Rich Plasma (PRP), exosomes, and Hydrafacial™ Keravive™ have shown immense potential in treating various types of hair loss by enhancing the scalp environment, stimulating follicular activity, and promoting cellular communication. These treatments focus on utilising the body's natural healing mechanisms to revive dormant follicles and encourage new growth.

1. **Platelet-Rich Plasma (PRP)**: PRP is a concentration of platelets derived from the patient's own blood, rich in growth factors that can enhance blood supply to hair follicles, stimulate cellular repair, and improve hair density.

2. **Exosome Therapy**: Exosomes are tiny vesicles that carry proteins, growth factors, and genetic material to nearby cells, facilitating intercellular communication and promoting tissue regeneration.

3. **Hydrafacial™ Keravive™**: This unique scalp treatment combines deep cleansing, hydration, and nourishment to create an optimal environment for hair growth. By removing dead skin cells and impurities and infusing the scalp with growth factors and peptides, Keravive™ enhances circulation and scalp health.

Integrating Nutritional Strategies and Lifestyle Optimisation

Optimal hair health is closely linked to nutritional status. Deficiencies in key nutrients like biotin, zinc, vitamin D, and iron can contribute to hair thinning and loss. Incorporating a diet rich in these nutrients can improve hair quality and promote regrowth. Additionally, lifestyle factors such as managing stress, getting adequate sleep, and maintaining a healthy scalp environment are crucial components of a comprehensive hair health strategy.

The Role of Ancestral Wisdom: Ayurveda and Traditional Chinese Medicine

While modern science has brought us sophisticated therapies, there is also wisdom to be gained from ancient traditions like Ayurveda and Traditional Chinese Medicine (TCM). Both Ayurveda and TCM view hair as a reflection of internal balance and believe that imbalances in organs like the liver or kidneys can manifest as hair loss. Herbs such as amla, bhringraj, He Shou Wu, and ginseng have been used for centuries to strengthen hair, nourish the scalp, and address systemic imbalances that contribute to hair loss.

Integrating these ancestral practices with modern science provides a comprehensive, individualised approach to hair health that addresses both internal and external factors.

Creating a Synergistic Approach to Hair Regeneration

The most effective hair restoration plans combine the best of modern science and traditional wisdom. This book provides evidence-based guidance on how to create personalised treatment plans that address the multifactorial nature of hair loss. It covers everything from optimising nutrition and hormonal health to incorporating advanced regenerative therapies and traditional remedies.

Whether you are a healthcare professional looking to expand your understanding of hair regeneration or an individual seeking to restore your hair's vitality, *From Thinning to Thriving: The Definitive Guide to Hair Restoration, Nutrition, and Advanced Therapies* will serve as your comprehensive resource. It is time to move beyond quick fixes and embrace a holistic approach that considers the intricate relationship between hair health and overall wellness.

The Journey Ahead

This book will guide you through the science and art of hair restoration, covering every aspect, from diagnostics and testing to the latest regenerative therapies and holistic strategies. Each chapter builds upon the next, providing practical insights and real-world case studies to illustrate the principles discussed.

Let us follow this journey, transforming thinning hair into thriving hair and reclaiming confidence and vitality along the way.

Summary: Introduction

Embracing a New Approach to Hair Restoration

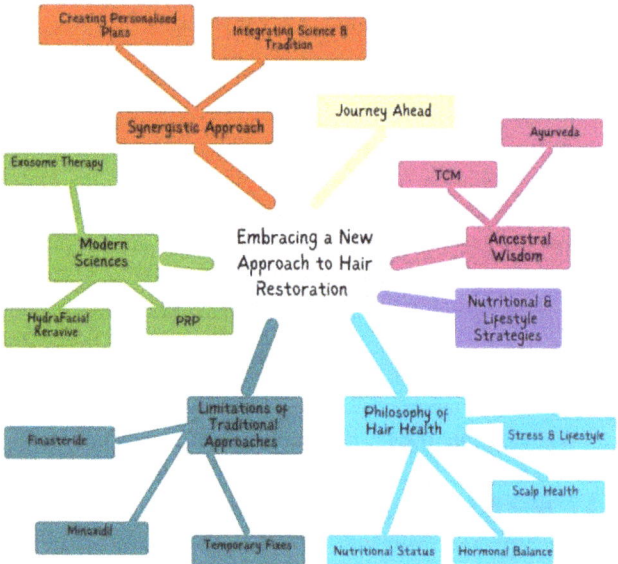

Chapter 1
Understanding Hair Health and Regeneration

1.1 The Hair Growth Cycle

Hair growth is a dynamic process governed by a complex cycle that consists of three primary phases: anagen, catagen, and telogen. Each phase plays a crucial role in determining hair density, length, and overall quality. Disruptions to this cycle can result in hair thinning, excessive shedding, or even permanent hair loss.

- **Anagen Phase (Growth Phase)**: The anagen phase is the active growth period for hair follicles and can last anywhere from 2 to 6 years, depending on genetics and overall health. During this phase, cells in the hair bulb rapidly divide, pushing the hair shaft upward and out of the scalp. Approximately 85-90% of the hair on a healthy scalp is in the anagen phase at any given time. Factors such as age, nutrition, and genetics determine the length of this phase. When the anagen phase is shortened, the hair may appear finer and more susceptible to falling out.

- **Catagen Phase (Transitional Phase)**: The catagen phase is a brief period that lasts about 2-3 weeks. It marks the end of active hair growth and is characterised by the detachment of the hair bulb from the blood supply. During this phase, hair follicles shrink and undergo structural changes, which prepare the hair to enter the resting phase. Only about 1-2% of hair is in the catagen phase at any time.

- **Telogen Phase (Resting and Shedding Phase)**: The telogen phase is a resting period that lasts around 3 months. During this phase, hair remains in the follicle without growing until it eventually sheds and a new anagen phase begins. This natural shedding process allows for new hair to replace old hair. Typically, 10-15% of hair is in the telogen phase at any given time. An increase in the percentage of hair in this phase can lead to noticeable hair thinning.

Factors Influencing Hair Growth and Density

The length and quality of each phase can be influenced by numerous factors, including genetics, hormonal balance, nutrition, and environmental exposures. Hormones such as oestrogen and testosterone play a critical role in regulating the growth cycle. For instance, elevated levels of dihydrotestosterone (DHT) can shorten the anagen phase, leading to thinner hair shafts. Nutritional factors like iron, biotin, and protein intake are also essential, as deficiencies in these nutrients can disrupt hair growth.

External factors such as ultraviolet (UV) radiation, chemical treatments, and pollutants can damage hair structure, causing breakage and weakening the hair shaft. Proper scalp care and minimising exposure to damaging factors can help maintain a balanced hair growth cycle.

1.2 Mechanisms of Hair Loss

Hair loss is a multifactorial condition with various underlying mechanisms that differ depending on the type of hair loss. Understanding these mechanisms is crucial for developing effective treatment strategies.

Androgenetic Alopecia (AGA)

Androgenetic alopecia, also known as male or female pattern baldness, is the most common form of hair loss. It is characterised by a progressive miniaturisation of hair follicles due to genetic predisposition and heightened sensitivity to DHT. In AGA, hair follicles shrink over time, leading to shorter, thinner hair until the follicles eventually become dormant. This condition often presents as a receding hairline and thinning crown in men and diffuse thinning across the scalp in women.

- **Genetic Predisposition**: AGA is inherited and follows a polygenic pattern, meaning multiple genes contribute to its development. The androgen receptor (AR) gene on the X chromosome has been identified as one of the key genetic markers associated with AGA.

- **Hormonal Influences**: DHT, a potent metabolite of testosterone, binds to androgen receptors in hair follicles, initiating a process that reduces hair follicle size and disrupts the growth cycle. In women, hormonal imbalances such as elevated androgens or decreased oestrogen levels can contribute to female pattern hair loss.

Telogen Effluvium (TE)

Telogen effluvium is characterised by an increased number of hair follicles entering the telogen (resting) phase prematurely. This results in diffuse thinning and increased hair shedding. TE can be triggered by physical or emotional stress, nutritional deficiencies, or systemic health conditions.

- **Stress and Telogen Effluvium**: Acute stress, illness, or surgical procedures can shock hair follicles into the resting phase, causing a sudden increase in shedding several weeks to months after the event. While TE is often reversible, it can become chronic if the underlying stressor is not addressed.

- **Nutritional Deficiencies**: Deficiencies in essential nutrients such as iron, zinc, vitamin D, and protein can impair hair growth and trigger TE. Restoring these nutrients often helps reverse the condition.

Alopecia Areata (AA)

Alopecia areata is an autoimmune disorder where the body's immune system mistakenly attacks hair follicles, resulting in patchy hair loss. The condition is characterised by the sudden onset of round, smooth patches of hair loss, and in severe cases, it can progress to total hair loss on the scalp (alopecia totalis) or entire body (alopecia universalis).

- **Autoimmune Mechanism**: In AA, T-lymphocytes (immune cells) target hair follicles as if they were foreign invaders. This autoimmune response leads to inflammation and disruption of the normal hair growth cycle. The exact cause of AA is unknown, but it is believed to involve a combination of genetic susceptibility and environmental triggers.

Role of Oxidative Stress and Environmental Toxins

Oxidative stress, caused by an imbalance between free radicals and antioxidants in the body, can damage hair follicle cells, leading to premature ageing and hair thinning. Environmental toxins such as pollution, heavy metals, and UV radiation exacerbate oxidative stress, contributing to hair follicle dysfunction.

Understanding the Mechanisms of Hair Loss

By identifying the specific mechanisms behind each type of hair loss, targeted treatment strategies can be developed. For example, anti-androgenic therapies such as Finasteride or topical DHT blockers are effective for androgenetic alopecia, while immune-modulating treatments like corticosteroids or biologics are used for alopecia areata.

1.3 The Science of Hair Regeneration

Hair regeneration is a rapidly evolving field that leverages the body's natural healing mechanisms to promote hair growth. Understanding the cellular and molecular processes involved in hair regeneration is key to developing effective therapeutic interventions.

Cellular Signalling Pathways in Hair Regeneration

Hair follicles are unique in that they undergo cycles of growth, regression, and rest. This cyclical nature is regulated by a complex interplay of signalling pathways, including:

- **Wnt/β-catenin Pathway**: Activation of the Wnt/β-catenin pathway is crucial for initiating the anagen (growth) phase. This pathway promotes the proliferation of hair follicle stem cells and enhances the expression of genes involved in hair growth.

- **Sonic Hedgehog (Shh) Pathway**: The Shh pathway plays a role in the development and maintenance of hair follicles. Modulating this pathway has been shown to stimulate hair regrowth in preclinical studies.

- **Growth Factors and Cytokines**: Growth factors such as platelet-derived growth factor (PDGF), fibroblast growth factor (FGF), and insulin-like growth factor (IGF) promote cellular proliferation and survival. Cytokines like interleukin-1 (IL-1) and tumour necrosis factor-alpha (TNF-α) can either support or inhibit hair growth, depending on the context.

Mechanisms of Action for Regenerative Therapies

Regenerative therapies aim to restore hair growth by modulating these signalling pathways and creating an optimal environment for hair follicle regeneration. Key therapies include:

- **Platelet-Rich Plasma (PRP)**: PRP contains a high concentration of growth factors that enhance cellular repair, stimulate angiogenesis (formation of new blood vessels), and prolong the anagen phase of hair growth. When injected into the scalp, PRP releases these growth factors, promoting the proliferation of dermal papilla cells and improving hair density.

- **Exosome Therapy**: Exosomes are nano-sized vesicles derived from stem cells that carry proteins, lipids, and genetic material to recipient cells. Exosome therapy enhances cellular communication and has shown promise in regenerating hair follicles and reducing inflammation.

- **Stem Cell Therapy**: Stem cells have the ability to differentiate into various cell types, making them ideal candidates for tissue regeneration. In hair restoration, stem cells are used to replenish damaged hair follicle cells and stimulate the growth of new follicles.

High Innovation in Hair Regeneration: Novel Agents and Therapies

Emerging therapies such as topical melatonin, peptides like GHK-Cu, and other novel agents are being explored for their ability to promote hair growth through unique mechanisms:

- **Melatonin**: Melatonin has antioxidant properties and modulates the hair growth cycle by promoting the anagen phase. It also reduces oxidative stress in hair follicles, making it an effective treatment for androgenetic alopecia and telogen effluvium.

- **Peptide Therapy**: Peptides such as GHK-Cu (a copper peptide) promote wound healing, reduce inflammation, and stimulate hair follicle cells. Peptide-based therapies are being developed as topical solutions to enhance hair growth and improve scalp health.

Conclusion

The science of hair regeneration is complex and multifaceted, involving a deep understanding of cellular signalling, growth factors, and regenerative therapies. By leveraging these mechanisms, it is possible to develop more effective strategies for treating various forms of hair loss and promoting hair health.

Summary: Understanding Hair Health and Regeneration

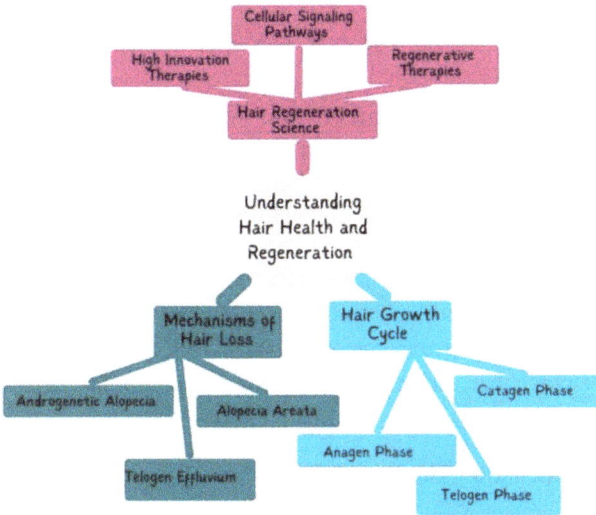

Chapter 2
Best Practices in Hair Regeneration: A Holistic Approach

2.1 Developing a Comprehensive Treatment Plan

A successful hair regeneration strategy begins with a comprehensive evaluation of the individual's unique health status, hair loss patterns, and lifestyle factors. Developing a personalised treatment plan involves more than just choosing a therapy—it requires a holistic assessment that addresses all underlying contributors to hair thinning or shedding. This section outlines the key factors that should be considered when formulating a hair restoration plan.

1. Understanding the Root Causes

Hair loss can stem from various root causes, including nutritional deficiencies, hormonal imbalances, stress, and systemic health issues. Therefore, the first step in creating an effective treatment plan is a thorough assessment, which should include a detailed patient history, visual inspection of the scalp, and appropriate diagnostic tests. Understanding these root causes enables practitioners to develop targeted treatment strategies that address the specific needs of each patient.

- **Hormonal Health**: For conditions like androgenetic alopecia, hormonal evaluation is crucial. Assessing levels of DHT, testosterone, oestrogen, and thyroid hormones provides insight into potential hormonal contributors to hair thinning. Anti-androgen therapies or hormonal modulation can be incorporated into the plan when necessary.

- **Nutritional Status**: Nutritional deficiencies, particularly in iron, vitamin D, zinc, and B vitamins, are common in patients with diffuse thinning or telogen effluvium. A comprehensive blood panel should assess these parameters to identify and correct any deficiencies.

- **Lifestyle Factors**: Chronic stress, poor sleep, and unhealthy dietary habits can significantly impact hair health. Integrating stress management techniques, sleep optimisation, and dietary interventions can improve the overall effectiveness of hair restoration therapies.

2. Setting Realistic Goals and Expectations

It is essential to set realistic goals and expectations for the patient. Hair regeneration is a gradual process, and significant improvement may take several months. Depending on the severity and type of hair loss, some patients may only experience stabilisation rather than regrowth, particularly in cases of advanced androgenetic alopecia. Discussing these expectations upfront helps build trust and ensures that patients remain committed to their treatment plan.

3. Multimodal Treatment Approach

Combining various therapeutic modalities often yields the best results in hair restoration. A multimodal approach integrates different therapies that complement each other, addressing multiple aspects of hair health simultaneously.

- **Topical Therapies**: These include Minoxidil, topical peptides, and melatonin. Topicals are particularly useful in maintaining scalp health and enhancing follicular activity.

- **Oral Supplements and Medications**: Oral supplements like biotin, vitamin D, iron, and saw palmetto support internal hair health, while medications such as Finasteride or Dutasteride help modulate hormone levels.

- **Regenerative Therapies**: Treatments like PRP, microneedling, and exosome therapy can stimulate dormant follicles and improve scalp health. Integrating these therapies into a treatment plan can enhance the efficacy of traditional methods.

4. Regular Monitoring and Adjustments

Hair growth is a dynamic process that requires ongoing monitoring. Regular follow-ups should be scheduled every three to six months to assess progress, make necessary adjustments to the treatment plan, and address any concerns. Modifications to the plan may include changing dosages of supplements, adding new therapies, or discontinuing treatments that aren't producing desired results.

2.2 Diagnostic and Testing Protocols

Diagnostic testing is an essential component of any hair restoration plan. It provides valuable insights into the underlying factors contributing to hair loss and helps guide therapeutic decisions. The following tests are commonly used in diagnosing and treating hair loss:

1. Blood Tests for Nutritional Deficiencies and Hormonal Imbalances

Comprehensive blood tests can identify nutritional deficiencies and hormonal imbalances that may be affecting hair health. Recommended blood tests include:

- **Complete Blood Count (CBC)**: Assesses overall health and identifies conditions like anaemia, which can contribute to hair loss.

- **Ferritin and Iron Levels**: Low iron stores are a common cause of telogen effluvium, particularly in women.

- **Thyroid Function Tests (TSH, T3, T4)**: Thyroid imbalances can disrupt the hair growth cycle and cause diffuse thinning.

- **Vitamin D3**: Deficiency in vitamin D is associated with several forms of hair loss, including alopecia areata and androgenetic alopecia.

- **Hormone Panel (DHT, Testosterone, SHBG, Estradiol)**: Evaluating androgen levels and hormonal balance is crucial in diagnosing androgenetic alopecia and determining the appropriate hormonal therapies.

2. Genetic Testing for Personalised Treatment Plans

Genetic testing, such as the Fagron TrichoTest™, can provide insight into genetic predispositions to hair loss. This test analyses variations in genes related to hair growth and the metabolism of drugs like Finasteride and Minoxidil. By identifying these genetic markers, practitioners can tailor treatment plans to optimise effectiveness and minimise side effects.

3. Scalp Biopsy and Trichoscopy

In cases where the diagnosis is unclear, a scalp biopsy can provide definitive information about the health of hair follicles and identify conditions like scarring alopecia. Trichoscopy, a non-invasive technique that uses magnification to visualise the scalp and hair shafts, can help detect the miniaturisation of follicles and differentiate between different types of alopecia.

4. Hair Pull Test and Wash Test

These clinical tests help quantify hair shedding. In the hair pull test, several strands of hair are gently pulled to determine if excessive shedding is occurring. The wash test involves washing hair over a defined period and counting the number of hairs shed.

2.3 Tailoring Treatments to Individual Needs

Effective hair restoration requires personalised treatment plans based on diagnostic results, patient history, and individual needs. This section provides a step-by-step guide to tailoring treatments.

1. Matching Therapies to the Type of Hair Loss

- **Androgenetic Alopecia**: Treatment typically involves DHT blockers like Finasteride, topical Minoxidil, and regenerative therapies like PRP or microneedling. Combining these therapies can enhance follicular activity and slow the progression of hair thinning.

- **Telogen Effluvium**: The focus should be on identifying and eliminating triggers, such as stress or nutritional deficiencies. Supplementation with iron, vitamin D, and B vitamins, along with stress management strategies, can support recovery.

- **Alopecia Areata**: Immune-modulating therapies like corticosteroids, topical immunotherapy, and JAK inhibitors may be considered. Regenerative therapies such as PRP or exosome therapy can also be integrated to support follicular health.

2. Choosing the Right Regenerative Therapies

- **Platelet-Rich Plasma (PRP)**: Best suited for patients with early-stage hair loss or those looking to enhance hair transplant results. PRP is effective for improving hair density and slowing the progression of thinning.

- **Exosome Therapy**: Recommended for individuals seeking cutting-edge treatment options. Exosomes can stimulate cellular communication, reduce inflammation, and promote hair growth.

- **Hydrafacial™ Keravive™**: Ideal for individuals with scalp issues such as dandruff, dryness, or poor circulation. This therapy combines cleansing, hydration, and infusion of growth factors and peptides to create a healthier scalp environment, enhancing the efficacy of other treatments.

3. Adjusting Treatment Plans Over Time

Hair restoration is a long-term commitment. As the patient's condition evolves, so too should the treatment plan. Adjustments may include:

- Switching from aggressive treatments to maintenance therapies as hair stabilises.

- Adding new therapies if progress plateaus.

- Modifying dosages of supplements or medications based on blood test results.

4. Integrating Lifestyle and Nutritional Support

Lifestyle factors such as diet, exercise, and stress management play a crucial role in supporting hair health. Tailoring nutritional advice and integrating supplements like biotin, iron, and omega-3 fatty acids can complement therapeutic interventions. Stress management techniques, such as mindfulness, yoga, and adaptogenic herbs, can reduce cortisol levels and support healthy hair growth.

Conclusion

Creating a comprehensive treatment plan for hair regeneration involves understanding the root causes of hair loss, utilising appropriate diagnostic tests, and tailoring therapies to the individual's unique needs. A multimodal approach that integrates topical treatments, regenerative therapies, and lifestyle optimisation is often the most effective strategy for restoring hair health and achieving long-term success.

Summary: Best Practices in Hair Regeneration: A Holistic Approach

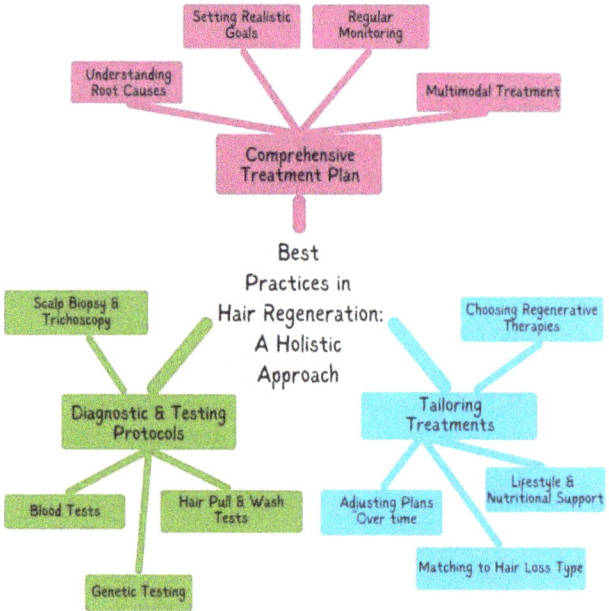

Chapter 3
Modern Regenerative Therapies for Hair Health

Modern regenerative therapies offer promising solutions for hair restoration by leveraging the body's natural healing mechanisms and utilising advanced technologies to optimise hair growth and follicular health. This chapter delves into key regenerative therapies such as Platelet-Rich Plasma (PRP), Carboxytherapy, Exosome Therapy, and advanced technologies like low-level laser therapy (LLLT), Hydrafacial™ Keravive™, and microneedling. Understanding how these therapies work, their benefits and best practices can help practitioners and patients achieve optimal outcomes in hair health.

3.1 Platelet-Rich Plasma (PRP) and Carboxytherapy

Mechanism of Action: How PRP Stimulates Follicle Activity and Promotes Growth

Platelet-Rich Plasma (PRP) therapy is a regenerative treatment that utilises the patient's own blood to extract a concentration of platelets rich in growth factors. These growth factors play a crucial role in stimulating cellular repair, increasing blood supply to hair follicles, and prolonging the anagen (growth) phase of the hair cycle. The process involves drawing a small amount of blood from the patient, processing it in a centrifuge to isolate the platelet-rich fraction, and injecting this plasma into the scalp.

PRP enhances follicular activity by:

1. **Stimulating Angiogenesis**: Growth factors such as vascular endothelial growth factor (VEGF) promote the formation of new blood vessels, improving blood supply to hair follicles and enhancing nutrient delivery.

2. **Encouraging Cellular Proliferation**: Platelet-derived growth factor (PDGF) and epidermal growth factor (EGF) stimulate the proliferation of dermal papilla cells, which are key in hair follicle development and maintenance.

3. **Reducing Inflammation**: PRP contains anti-inflammatory cytokines that can reduce scalp inflammation, creating a healthier environment for hair growth.

Combined Effect of Carboxytherapy on Enhancing Blood Flow and Oxygenation

Carboxytherapy involves the infusion of medical-grade carbon dioxide (CO_2) gas into the scalp. The body responds to this influx of CO_2 by increasing blood flow to the area, thereby enhancing oxygen delivery and nutrient supply to the hair follicles. When combined with PRP, carboxytherapy can amplify the results by promoting better absorption of growth factors and improving overall scalp health.

Best Practices and Case Studies

PRP and carboxytherapy are most effective when used in combination. The recommended protocol involves three sessions of PRP therapy spaced four to six weeks apart, with carboxytherapy applied concurrently. This combination therapy has shown significant results in patients with androgenetic alopecia, telogen effluvium, and alopecia areata.

Case Study: John, a 45-year-old male with early-stage androgenetic alopecia, underwent a series of PRP and carboxytherapy treatments. After three sessions, he reported a noticeable increase in hair density and reduced hair shedding. His results continued to improve over the next six months, with maintenance sessions every three months.

3.2 Exosome Therapy for Hair Regeneration

What Are Exosomes? Their Role in Cellular Communication and Repair

Exosomes are extracellular vesicles derived from stem cells that contain proteins, lipids, and genetic material. They function as messengers between cells, facilitating intercellular communication and promoting cellular repair and regeneration. Exosome therapy involves injecting these vesicles into the scalp, where they deliver growth factors and cytokines that activate dormant hair follicles, reduce inflammation, and promote hair regrowth.

Comparing Exosome Therapy to Traditional Stem Cell Therapy

While traditional stem cell therapy utilises the entire stem cell to promote regeneration, exosome therapy uses only the vesicles secreted by these cells. This makes exosome therapy a less invasive and more efficient option, as the vesicles can be absorbed more readily by recipient cells. Moreover, exosome therapy poses a lower risk of immune rejection and has shown promising results in hair restoration without the need for extracting or harvesting stem cells from the patient.

Outcomes and Patient Experiences with Exosome-Based Treatments

Exosome therapy has been shown to increase hair density, improve hair thickness, and promote overall scalp health. It is particularly beneficial for patients who have not responded to traditional therapies or are looking for a cutting-edge, minimally invasive solution.

Case Study: Sarah, a 50-year-old female experiencing diffuse thinning due to chronic stress, received a series of exosome injections. After four months, she reported a 30% increase in hair density and a significant reduction in hair shedding. Her results were maintained with bi-annual booster sessions.

3.3 Advanced Technologies: Laser Therapy, Hydrafacial™ Keravive™, and Microneedling

Laser Therapy: Role of Low-Level Laser Therapy (LLLT) in Stimulating Dormant Follicles and Enhancing Cellular Energy

Low-Level Laser Therapy (LLLT) is a non-invasive treatment that uses red and near-infrared light to penetrate the scalp and stimulate hair follicles. LLLT enhances mitochondrial function in cells, increasing ATP production and promoting cellular energy. This leads to improved follicle function, reduced inflammation, and prolonged anagen phase.

- **Mechanism of Action**: LLLT works by emitting specific wavelengths of light that are absorbed by chromophores in the hair follicle cells. This stimulates cellular respiration and activates pathways that lead to hair growth.

- **Benefits**: LLLT has been shown to increase hair density and thickness, improve scalp health, and reduce the rate of hair loss. It is particularly effective when used in conjunction with other regenerative therapies like PRP or topical treatments.

Case Study: David, a 40-year-old male with androgenetic alopecia, used a home LLLT device along with topical Minoxidil. After six months, he experienced a 25% increase in hair density and reduced visibility of his scalp.

Hydrafacial™ Keravive™: Combining Exfoliation, Hydration, and Nourishment for a Healthy Scalp

Hydrafacial™ Keravive™ is a scalp-focused therapy that involves a three-step process of cleansing, hydration, and infusion of growth factors and peptides. It is designed to create an optimal environment for hair growth by addressing scalp issues such as dryness, clogged follicles, and poor circulation.

- **Mechanism of Action**: The first step involves a deep cleansing and exfoliation to remove dead skin cells, excess oil, and impurities. The second step infuses the scalp with a hydrating serum containing growth factors, peptides, and other nutrients. The final step involves a take-home spray that helps maintain hydration and nourishment between treatments.

- **Benefits**: Hydrafacial™ Keravive™ improves scalp health, reduces inflammation, enhances microcirculation, and promotes the absorption of other topical treatments. It can be used as a standalone treatment or combined with other therapies like PRP or microneedling to enhance results.

- **Best Practices**: For optimal results, three sessions spaced four weeks apart are recommended, followed by maintenance sessions every three months.

Case Study: Linda, a 35-year-old female with a history of dry, flaky scalp, underwent a series of Hydrafacial™ Keravive™ treatments. After three sessions, she reported improved scalp hydration, reduced flakiness, and increased hair density. The combination of Hydrafacial™ Keravive™ and PRP therapy further enhanced her hair health and appearance.

Microneedling: Creating Micro-Injuries to Activate Growth Factors and Improve Topical Absorption

Microneedling, also known as collagen induction therapy, involves creating controlled micro-injuries on the scalp using a device with fine needles. These micro-injuries stimulate the body's wound-healing response, promoting collagen production and increasing the absorption of topical treatments.

- **Mechanism of Action**: The micro-injuries trigger the release of growth factors and cytokines that stimulate hair follicle stem cells. Microneedling also improves blood flow to the scalp and enhances the penetration of topical agents like PRP, Minoxidil, or peptides.

- **Benefits**: Microneedling is effective in improving hair density, reducing hair thinning, and enhancing the results of other therapies. It can be used alone or in combination with PRP, exosomes, or topical treatments.

- **Combination Therapies**: Microneedling is often paired with PRP or exosomes to boost their absorption and efficacy. The micro-channels created by microneedling allow these regenerative agents to reach deeper layers of the scalp, maximising their impact.

Case Study: Mark, a 42-year-old male with early-stage hair loss, received microneedling sessions combined with PRP every six weeks. After five sessions, he saw a marked improvement in hair density and reduced hairline recession. He continued with maintenance sessions every three months to sustain his results.

Choosing the Right Advanced Technology for Your Needs

When selecting advanced technologies for hair regeneration, consider the following factors:

- **Type and Stage of Hair Loss**: LLLT is ideal for early-stage hair loss, while Hydrafacial™ Keravive™ is beneficial for improving scalp health in patients with dry or inflamed scalps. Microneedling is effective for individuals looking to enhance the absorption of other treatments.

- **Patient Preferences and Comfort**: Some patients may prefer non-invasive treatments like LLLT, while others may be open to more intensive therapies like microneedling or PRP.

- **Combination Approaches**: For best results, consider combining these advanced technologies with other regenerative therapies to address multiple aspects of hair health.

Conclusion

Modern regenerative therapies offer a powerful suite of options for treating hair loss and promoting hair health. From the stimulating effects of PRP and carboxytherapy to the cutting-edge benefits of exosomes and advanced technologies like LLLT, Hydrafacial™ Keravive™, and microneedling, these therapies represent the forefront of hair restoration. Integrating these modalities into a comprehensive treatment plan can optimise hair growth, restore confidence, and support overall scalp health.

Summary: Modern Regenerative Therapies for Hair Health

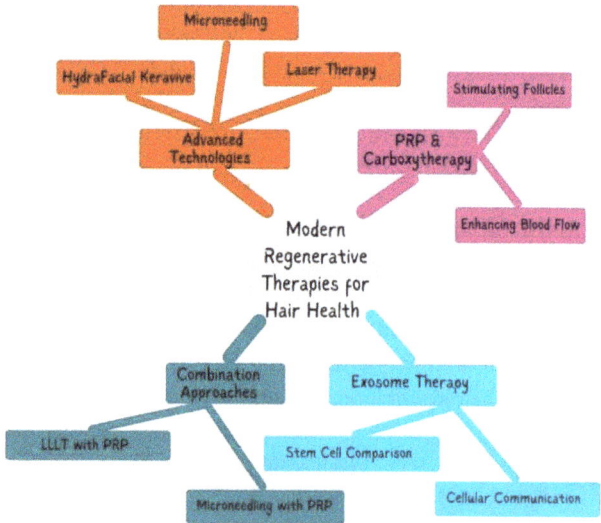

Chapter 4
Hair Transplant Innovations and Best Practices

Hair transplantation has advanced significantly over the last decade, moving from traditional strip excision techniques to more refined methods like Follicular Unit Extraction (FUE) and the integration of regenerative therapies. This chapter explores the latest innovations in hair transplant technology, outlines best practices for achieving optimal results, and discusses how combining transplants with regenerative therapies like PRP and exosomes can significantly improve outcomes.

4.1 Innovations in Hair Transplant Technology

Hair transplantation involves moving healthy hair follicles from a donor site—typically the back or sides of the head—to an area of thinning or baldness. The goal is to restore natural hair density, improve the hairline, and enhance overall appearance. There are two primary techniques for hair transplantation: Follicular Unit Transplantation (FUT) and Follicular Unit Extraction (FUE). While both methods have their advantages, recent innovations have further refined these techniques, making hair transplantation more efficient and less invasive.

FUE (Follicular Unit Extraction) vs. FUT (Follicular Unit Transplantation)

- **FUE** involves extracting individual hair follicles from the donor area using a small, circular punch. Each follicle is then implanted into the recipient site. This method leaves minimal scarring and allows for a quicker recovery. FUE is ideal for patients seeking a less invasive option or those who prefer to wear their hair short.

- **FUT** involves removing a strip of scalp tissue from the donor area, dissecting it into individual follicular units, and implanting them into the recipient site. While FUT can harvest a larger number of grafts in a single session, it leaves a linear scar on the donor site, which may be visible if the hair is cut very short.

The Role of Robotic Assistance in Hair Transplantation

Robotic technology, such as the ARTAS® Robotic Hair Transplant System, has revolutionised hair transplantation by automating the FUE process. Robotic systems use artificial intelligence to identify the healthiest follicles for extraction and implant them with precision, minimising human error and reducing the risk of follicular damage.

- **Advantages of Robotic Hair Transplants**: Enhanced accuracy in graft extraction and placement, reduced transaction rates (damage to follicles during extraction), and faster procedural times.

- **Patient Suitability**: Robotic hair transplantation is particularly beneficial for individuals with high follicular density in the donor area and those seeking to maximise the efficiency of their procedure.

Integration of Regenerative Therapies in Transplant Recovery and Optimisation

The use of regenerative therapies such as PRP, exosomes, and stem cells has become a cornerstone in optimising hair transplant outcomes. These therapies enhance graft survival, accelerate healing, and promote new hair growth in both the transplanted and surrounding areas.

- **PRP Therapy**: PRP is often applied to the recipient area immediately after graft implantation. The growth factors in

PRP promote faster wound healing and improve graft anchoring and survival.

- **Exosome Therapy**: Exosomes deliver signalling molecules that enhance cellular repair and reduce inflammation, making them an ideal adjunctive therapy for post-transplant recovery.

- **Stem Cell Therapy**: Stem cells can differentiate into various cell types, promoting tissue repair and regeneration. Incorporating stem cell therapy into transplant protocols can enhance overall follicular health and density.

Emerging Innovations in Hair Transplantation

Innovations such as long-hair FUE (where the patient's hair is not shaved before the procedure), beard and body hair transplants, and the use of bioengineered scaffolds to support graft growth are pushing the boundaries of what hair transplantation can achieve. As these technologies evolve, they will continue to expand the possibilities for restoring hair in individuals with advanced hair loss.

4.2 Best Practices for Hair Transplantation

Achieving the best results from hair transplantation requires careful planning, pre-operative preparation, and meticulous post-operative care. This section outlines the best practices to optimise transplant outcomes and ensure long-term success.

Pre-Transplant Preparation: Optimising Scalp and Follicular Health

Preparing the scalp for transplantation is crucial for maximising graft survival and ensuring the overall health of the transplanted area. Pre-transplant preparation may include:

1. **Scalp Conditioning**: Using topical treatments like Minoxidil or peptides to improve blood circulation and create a healthier scalp environment.

2. **Nutritional Support**: Supplementing with vitamins such as biotin, vitamin D, zinc, and iron to support follicular health and reduce the risk of shedding.

3. **PRP or Exosome Therapy**: Administering PRP or exosomes a few weeks before the transplant can precondition the scalp, enhancing the overall health of the recipient area.

Post-Transplant Care: Nutritional Support, Scalp Care, and Novel Therapies like Melatonin

Proper post-transplant care is essential for graft survival and successful hair regrowth. Recommendations include:

1. **Nutritional Support**: Continuing with supplements like biotin, vitamin D, and omega-3 fatty acids to support hair health. Additionally, incorporating amino acids like L-cysteine and taurine can enhance keratin production and follicle strength.

2. **Scalp Care**: Gentle cleansing of the scalp to prevent infection and promote healing. Avoiding harsh shampoos or products that can irritate the scalp is essential during the recovery phase.

3. **Melatonin Therapy**: Topical melatonin has been shown to extend the anagen phase and promote hair growth. Applying melatonin solutions, post-transplant can support hair density and improve the overall quality of new hair.

Common Challenges and How to Overcome Them

*   **Shock Loss**: Temporary shedding of transplanted and native hair following the procedure. Shock loss is common but usually resolves within a few months. Incorporating therapies like PRP or exosomes can help mitigate this.

- **Folliculitis**: Inflammation or infection of hair follicles can occur post-transplant. Using topical antibiotics and anti-inflammatory agents can help manage and prevent folliculitis.

- **Scarring**: Minimising scarring is critical, particularly in FUE procedures. Using post-surgical treatments like microneedling or silicone gels can reduce scar visibility and improve the aesthetic outcome.

4.3 Combining Hair Transplants with Regenerative Therapies

Integrating regenerative therapies with hair transplants can significantly enhance the results by promoting healing, improving graft survival, and encouraging new hair growth. This section explores the benefits of combining PRP, exosomes, stem cells, and other regenerative therapies with hair transplantation.

Using Regenerative Therapies Like PRP, Exosomes, and Novel Agents to Enhance Transplant Results

Regenerative therapies can be used at various stages of the transplant process:

1. **Pre-Operative**: Administering PRP or exosome therapy before the transplant can improve the health of both the donor and recipient sites. These therapies increase vascularity, reduce inflammation, and create a more supportive environment for graft implantation.

2. **Intra-Operative**: Applying PRP to the recipient area during the procedure helps prepare the scalp for graft placement, enhancing graft survival and reducing trauma to the follicles.

3. **Post-Operative**: Regular PRP or exosome sessions post-transplant accelerate healing, reduce inflammation, and stimulate the growth of both transplanted and surrounding native hair.

Role of Anti-Inflammatory Agents, Antioxidants, and Peptides in Post-Transplant Recovery

Incorporating anti-inflammatory agents and antioxidants can mitigate oxidative stress and reduce the risk of graft rejection or inflammation. Peptides like GHK-Cu (Copper Peptide) can promote collagen production and enhance tissue repair.

1. **Anti-Inflammatory Agents**: Topical corticosteroids, oral NSAIDs, or herbal agents like curcumin can help control inflammation post-transplant.

2. **Antioxidants**: Vitamins C and E, coenzyme Q_{10}, and resveratrol can reduce oxidative damage, support tissue repair, and improve overall scalp health.

3. **Peptide Therapy**: Peptides like GHK-Cu stimulate the production of extracellular matrix components, enhance wound healing, and promote hair follicle growth.

Case Studies Showcasing Successful Integration of Therapies

- **Case Study 1**: Michael, a 35-year-old male with a receding hairline and crown thinning, received an FUE transplant combined with PRP therapy. Pre- and post-operative PRP sessions enhanced graft survival, resulting in a 30% increase in hair density compared to his previous hair transplant procedure without PRP.

- **Case Study 2**: Anna, a 50-year-old female with diffuse thinning due to telogen effluvium, underwent a hair transplant combined with exosome therapy. Exosome injections significantly accelerated healing and minimised shock loss, leading to improved hair density and faster recovery.

Combining Hair Transplants with Topical and Oral Therapies for Long-Term Success

- **Topical Therapies**: Using Minoxidil or peptides like GHK-Cu can maintain the health of native hair and support the growth of transplanted hair.

- **Oral Therapies**: Oral anti-androgens like Finasteride or Dutasteride can prevent further hair loss in androgen-sensitive areas, stabilising the overall condition and supporting long-term success.

Integrating Multiple Modalities for Comprehensive Care

The best outcomes are achieved when hair transplants are combined with a comprehensive approach that includes nutritional support, hormonal modulation, and regenerative therapies. By addressing the multiple factors that contribute to hair loss, it is possible to create a synergistic effect that enhances overall hair health and maximises the benefits of hair transplantation.

Conclusion

Innovative hair transplant technologies and the integration of regenerative therapies have transformed the landscape of hair restoration. By combining surgical techniques like FUE and FUT with cutting-edge therapies like PRP, exosomes, and stem cells, practitioners can achieve exceptional results that were previously unattainable. These advances, coupled with best practices in pre- and post-transplant care, provide a comprehensive approach to hair restoration that is both effective and sustainable.

Summary: Hair Transplant Innovations and Best Practices

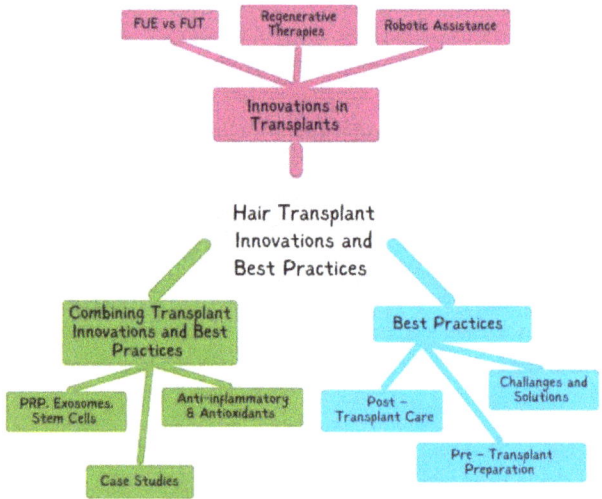

Chapter 5
The Role of Trichologists in Hair Health

Trichology is a specialised field dedicated to the scientific study of hair and scalp health. Trichologists play a pivotal role in diagnosing and managing hair disorders, bridging the gap between dermatology and hair restoration. With expertise in assessing hair and scalp conditions, trichologists provide valuable insights into the underlying causes of hair loss and contribute to developing comprehensive, individualised treatment plans. This chapter explores the scope of trichology, the diagnostic tools used by trichologists, and their integration into modern regenerative hair treatments.

5.1 What Is Trichology?

Overview of Trichology as a Scientific Discipline

Trichology is derived from the Greek word "trikhos," meaning hair, and "logos," meaning study. It is a branch of dermatology that focuses on the anatomy, biology, and pathology of hair and scalp health. Trichologists are professionals trained in recognising and treating conditions such as hair thinning, hair loss, dandruff, scalp inflammation, and various types of alopecia.

While trichology is not a licensed medical speciality in most countries, it plays a crucial role in hair restoration and health management. Trichologists possess an in-depth understanding of the hair growth cycle, hair structure, and factors that influence hair health, including genetics, nutrition, hormones, and environmental exposures. They are often the first point of contact for individuals experiencing hair and scalp issues, providing non-surgical and holistic approaches to treatment.

How Trichologists Differ from Dermatologists and Hair Transplant Surgeons

Trichologists, dermatologists, and hair transplant surgeons each have distinct roles in hair health:

- **Trichologists**: Specialise in the non-medical assessment and treatment of hair and scalp conditions. They focus on understanding the root causes of hair loss and developing non-invasive, holistic treatment plans. Trichologists use a variety of diagnostic tools, including trichoscopy, hair pull tests, and scalp biopsies, to identify the type and severity of hair loss.

- **Dermatologists**: Are medical doctors who specialise in diagnosing and treating skin, hair, and nail disorders. They have the authority to prescribe medications, perform biopsies, and provide advanced medical treatments for hair loss, such as corticosteroid injections for alopecia areata.

- **Hair Transplant Surgeons**: Are specialised surgeons who perform hair transplant procedures using techniques like Follicular Unit Extraction (FUE) or Follicular Unit Transplantation (FUT). Their focus is on surgically restoring hair density in areas of significant hair loss.

While trichologists do not perform surgical procedures or prescribe medications, they complement the work of dermatologists and hair transplant surgeons by providing pre- and post-treatment care, optimising scalp health, and supporting the overall success of hair restoration therapies.

When to See a Trichologist

Individuals should consider seeing a trichologist if they experience:

- Gradual or sudden hair thinning.

- Unexplained hair shedding.

- Scalp issues such as itching, flaking, or redness.

- Hair breakage or changes in hair texture.

Trichologists are particularly beneficial for individuals seeking a holistic, non-invasive approach to managing hair and scalp concerns. They can provide guidance on lifestyle modifications, dietary changes, and topical treatments to support hair health.

5.2 The Trichologist's Approach to Hair Loss

Conducting Detailed Hair and Scalp Assessments

Trichologists conduct comprehensive hair and scalp assessments to understand the nature and extent of hair loss. A typical assessment involves taking a detailed patient history, which includes questions about diet, lifestyle, family history, and any recent illnesses or stressors that may contribute to hair loss. This holistic approach helps identify potential triggers and underlying causes that may not be immediately obvious.

Diagnostic Tools Used by Trichologists

Trichologists employ a range of diagnostic tools to evaluate hair and scalp health:

1. **Trichoscopy**: A non-invasive diagnostic technique that uses a dermatoscope or digital trichoscope to magnify and visualise the scalp and hair shafts. Trichoscopy provides detailed images of the hair follicles, hair density, and scalp condition, helping to diagnose conditions such as androgenetic alopecia, telogen effluvium, and scalp psoriasis.

2. **Hair Pull Test**: Involves gently pulling a small section of hair to determine the number of hairs shed. An increased number of hairs shed may indicate telogen effluvium or other diffuse hair loss conditions.

3. **Wash Test**: A method used to quantify hair shedding. Patients are asked to collect shed hairs during a standard hair wash, and the number of hairs shed is analysed to assess the severity of hair loss.

4. **Scalp Biopsy**: While more commonly performed by dermatologists, trichologists may recommend a scalp biopsy in cases where the diagnosis is unclear or to differentiate between scarring and non-scarring alopecia.

5. **Microscopic Analysis**: Trichologists use microscopes to analyse hair shafts for structural abnormalities, such as thinning, breakage, or changes in pigmentation. This can help identify conditions like trichorrhexis nodosa or diagnose hair shaft disorders.

Developing a Personalised Treatment Plan

Based on the assessment and diagnostic results, trichologists develop personalised treatment plans tailored to the individual's specific condition. Treatment plans may include recommendations for dietary changes, stress management techniques, topical applications, and referrals to medical professionals if necessary. In cases of hair loss due to hormonal imbalances or systemic health issues, trichologists may work alongside endocrinologists or dermatologists to provide a comprehensive approach to care.

5.3 Integrating Trichology into Regenerative Hair Treatments

How Trichologists Collaborate with Other Professionals

Trichologists often collaborate with dermatologists, hair transplant surgeons, and regenerative medicine specialists to ensure a comprehensive approach to hair restoration. By sharing diagnostic findings and insights into the patient's scalp health, trichologists help optimise treatment outcomes.

- **Pre-Treatment Preparation**: Trichologists prepare the scalp for surgical or regenerative treatments by ensuring it is in optimal health. This may involve scalp conditioning, anti-inflammatory therapies, or addressing scalp conditions like dandruff or seborrheic dermatitis.

- **Post-Treatment Care**: After hair transplants or regenerative treatments like PRP or exosome therapy, trichologists provide ongoing care to promote healing, reduce inflammation, and support new hair growth. Post-treatment care may include regular scalp assessments, topical therapies, and guidance on maintaining a healthy scalp environment.

Role of Trichology in Pre- and Post-Treatment Care

Trichologists play a vital role in both pre- and post-treatment care for individuals undergoing hair transplantation or regenerative therapies. Their expertise in scalp health and hair care complements medical and surgical interventions, improving overall outcomes and patient satisfaction.

Pre-Treatment Care

1. **Scalp Health Optimisation**: Trichologists use treatments like microneedling, low-level laser therapy (LLLT), or topical applications to optimise scalp health before surgical or regenerative interventions. This preparation increases the likelihood of graft survival and enhances the overall success of the treatment.

2. **Nutritional and Lifestyle Guidance**: Addressing nutritional deficiencies and providing lifestyle recommendations to improve systemic health can enhance hair restoration outcomes.

Post-Treatment Care

1. **Monitoring and Maintenance**: Trichologists closely monitor the scalp and hair after treatment to detect any signs of complications, such as folliculitis, scarring, or shock loss. Early intervention can prevent minor issues from escalating and ensure a smooth recovery process.

2. **Supporting Hair Regrowth**: Trichologists use therapies like PRP, topical peptides, or LLLT to support hair regrowth and optimise the results of surgical or regenerative procedures. Regular follow-up visits and scalp assessments help track progress and make any necessary adjustments to the treatment plan.

Integrating Trichology into a Comprehensive Hair Health Strategy

Trichologists serve as an essential part of a multidisciplinary team dedicated to hair restoration. By focusing on scalp health, optimising treatment outcomes, and providing ongoing support, trichologists contribute significantly to the success of both non-invasive and surgical hair restoration therapies.

Conclusion

Trichologists play a unique and indispensable role in the field of hair health. Their expertise in diagnosing and managing hair and scalp disorders, combined with their collaborative approach to working with other professionals, makes them invaluable in the holistic management of hair loss. Integrating trichology into regenerative hair treatments not only improves treatment outcomes but also ensures long-term hair health and patient satisfaction.

Summary: The Role of Trichologists in Hair Health

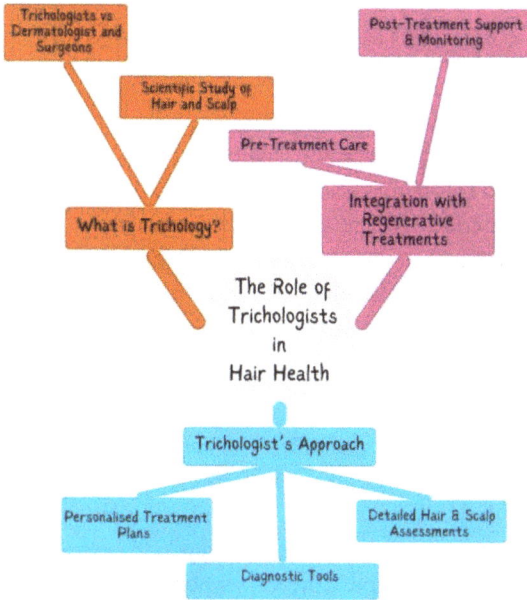

Chapter 6
Nutritional Strategies for Optimal Hair Health

Nutritional health is intrinsically linked to hair growth and quality. Deficiencies in certain vitamins, minerals, and macronutrients can contribute to hair thinning, loss, and poor hair quality. This chapter explores the critical role of nutrition in hair health, delves into the essential nutrients needed for optimal hair growth, and provides guidance on supplements and herbal options that can support hair regeneration and scalp health.

6.1 The Role of Diet in Hair Regeneration

Dietary intake plays a vital role in maintaining healthy hair and promoting hair growth. Hair follicles are metabolically active structures that require a constant supply of nutrients, and any deficiencies can disrupt the hair growth cycle. A balanced diet rich in proteins, vitamins, and minerals supports the structure of hair strands, the health of hair follicles, and the overall appearance of hair.

How Nutrients Affect Hair Growth

The hair growth cycle is divided into three phases: anagen (growth), catagen (transition), and telogen (resting). Optimal nutrition is required to sustain the anagen phase and ensure that hair remains in the growth stage for as long as possible. Nutritional deficiencies can shorten this phase, leading to increased hair shedding and slower regrowth.

- **Proteins and Amino Acids**: Hair is composed primarily of keratin, a fibrous protein made from amino acids. Sufficient dietary protein is essential for keratin synthesis, and amino acids like cysteine, methionine, and lysine play a key role in hair strength and elasticity.

- **Essential Fatty Acids**: Omega-3 and omega-6 fatty acids are critical for maintaining the scalp's lipid barrier, which protects hair follicles from environmental damage. They also have anti-inflammatory properties that can help reduce scalp inflammation, a common cause of hair thinning.

- **Vitamins and Minerals**: Vitamins such as A, C, D, and E, and minerals like iron, zinc, and magnesium are vital for hair follicle health and the prevention of hair loss. These nutrients act as cofactors in various enzymatic reactions within the hair follicle, supporting cellular turnover and metabolic activity.

Dietary Deficiencies and Their Impact on Hair Health

Certain deficiencies are particularly common among individuals experiencing hair loss:

- **Iron Deficiency**: Iron is a critical component of haemoglobin, which carries oxygen to hair follicles. Low iron levels can lead to anaemia, reduced oxygen delivery, and impaired hair growth. Women of childbearing age are especially at risk due to menstrual blood loss.

- **Zinc Deficiency**: Zinc is involved in protein synthesis and cellular division, making it essential for hair follicle function. Low zinc levels can lead to hair shedding, weakened hair structure, and reduced hair volume.

- **Vitamin D Deficiency**: Vitamin D plays a role in the creation of new hair follicles and the activation of follicular stem cells. Deficiency in this vitamin is associated with conditions like alopecia areata and telogen effluvium.

- **Protein Deficiency**: Insufficient protein intake can cause hair to enter the resting phase prematurely, leading to increased hair shedding. Vegans and vegetarians are at higher risk of protein deficiency, making it important to include adequate plant-based protein sources.

Balancing Your Diet for Optimal Hair Health

A balanced diet that includes a variety of nutrient-dense foods can support hair health:

- **Protein Sources**: Lean meats, poultry, fish, eggs, legumes, nuts, and seeds.

- **Healthy Fats**: Olive oil, avocados, nuts, seeds, and fatty fish like salmon.

- **Vitamins and Minerals**: Green leafy vegetables, citrus fruits, berries, nuts, and whole grains.

Incorporating a range of nutrient-rich foods ensures that the body receives the necessary components to sustain hair growth and reduce the risk of hair loss due to nutritional deficiencies.

6.2 Essential Nutrients for Hair Health

For hair to thrive, the body requires a range of vitamins, minerals, and other nutrients. The following nutrients are particularly crucial for maintaining healthy hair and promoting growth:

1. Vitamin D3

Vitamin D3 plays a crucial role in the proliferation of keratinocytes and hair follicle cycling. Deficiency in vitamin D is associated with hair loss conditions such as alopecia areata and telogen effluvium. High-dose vitamin D3 supplementation has been shown to promote hair growth by stimulating hair follicle cycling and reducing inflammation.

- **Sources**: Fatty fish (e.g., salmon, mackerel), fortified foods, and sunlight exposure.

- **Recommended Intake**: 2,000 to 4,000 IU daily or higher doses under medical supervision for those with a deficiency.

2. B Vitamins (Biotin, B6, B12)

B vitamins are vital for hair health, as they support cellular metabolism and energy production. Biotin (B7) strengthens hair by improving keratin structure, while B6 and B12 contribute to red blood cell formation and oxygen delivery to hair follicles.

- **Sources**: Eggs, dairy products, lean meats, whole grains, and leafy greens.

- **Recommended Intake**: Biotin—30 to 100 mcg daily; B6—1.3 to 2 mg daily; B12—2.4 mcg daily.

3. Vitamin A

Vitamin A regulates the production of sebum, an oily substance that moisturises the scalp and maintains hair health. However, excessive vitamin A intake can lead to hair loss, so it is important to maintain balanced levels.

- **Sources**: Carrots, sweet potatoes, spinach, and fortified cereals.

- **Recommended Intake**: 700 to 900 mcg daily.

4. Vitamin C

Vitamin C is a powerful antioxidant that helps protect hair follicles from oxidative stress. It also aids in the absorption of iron and supports collagen production, which is essential for hair structure.

- **Sources**: Citrus fruits, berries, kiwi, and bell peppers.

- **Recommended Intake**: 75 to 90 mg daily.

5. Iron

Iron deficiency is a leading cause of hair loss, particularly in women. It is essential for oxygen transport to hair follicles and overall follicular health.

- **Sources**: Red meat, poultry, seafood, lentils, and spinach.

- **Recommended Intake**: 8 to 18 mg daily, with higher doses under supervision for those with confirmed deficiencies.

6. Zinc

Zinc supports hair follicle health by regulating cell growth and repair. It also helps maintain the oil glands around the follicles, reducing the risk of dandruff and scalp irritation.

- **Sources**: Meat, shellfish, legumes, seeds, and nuts.

- **Recommended Intake**: 8 to 11 mg daily.

7. Magnesium

Magnesium is involved in over 300 enzymatic reactions in the body, including those that influence hair growth. It helps reduce stress, a common contributor to hair loss.

- **Sources**: Dark leafy greens, nuts, seeds, and whole grains.

- **Recommended Intake**: 310 to 420 mg daily.

8. Omega-3 and Omega-6 Fatty Acids

These essential fatty acids help reduce inflammation and support scalp health. They can prevent dry, brittle hair and promote overall hair vitality.

- **Sources**: Fatty fish, flaxseeds, chia seeds, and walnuts.

- **Recommended Intake**: 1,100 to 1,600 mg daily.

9. Copper Peptides

Copper peptides promote hair growth by increasing blood flow to the scalp and reducing follicle miniaturisation. They also play a role in the synthesis of melanin, which gives hair its colour.

- **Sources**: Liver, shellfish, nuts, and seeds.

- Recommended Intake: 900 mcg daily.

6.3 Supplements and Herbal Options

In addition to dietary sources, certain supplements and herbal remedies can enhance hair health and support the effectiveness of nutritional strategies.

Key Supplements for Hair Health

1. **Nanocelle Vitamin D3 + K2:** This combination supplement improves the absorption of vitamin D3 and supports bone health and hair follicle function. Vitamin K2 ensures that calcium is properly utilised, preventing calcification of the hair follicles.

   - **Dosage:** 1,000 to 5,000 IU of Vitamin D3 with 100 mcg of Vitamin K2 daily.

2. **Biotin and Collagen Peptides:** Biotin enhances keratin production, while collagen peptides support the structural integrity of the hair shaft. Together, these supplements strengthen hair and improve elasticity.

   - **Dosage:** Biotin—2,500 to 10,000 mcg daily; Collagen Peptides—5 to 10 grams daily.

3. **Omega-3 Fish Oil:** Fish oil supplements provide a concentrated source of omega-3 fatty acids, reducing scalp inflammation and supporting hair health.

   - **Dosage**: 1,000 to 2,000 mg daily.

4. **Saw Palmetto:** Saw palmetto is a natural DHT blocker that can reduce androgenic effects on hair follicles. It is particularly effective in cases of androgenetic alopecia.

   - **Dosage**: 320 mg daily of standardised extract.

Herbal Options for Hair Health

1. **Ashwagandha:** An adaptogenic herb, ashwagandha helps regulate cortisol levels and reduce stress-related hair loss.

   - **Dosage**: 300 to 500 mg of standardised extract daily.

2. **He Shou Wu (Fo-Ti):** A staple in Traditional Chinese Medicine, He Shou Wu is used to nourish the blood and support hair pigmentation and strength.

   - **Dosage**: 500 to 1,000 mg of root extract daily.

3. **Bhringraj:** An Ayurvedic herb known as the "King of Hair," Bhringraj supports scalp health and promotes hair growth.

   - **Dosage**: 500 mg of extract daily or applied topically as an oil.

Probiotics and Prebiotics for Scalp Health

The gut-skin axis plays a role in hair health, and maintaining a balanced gut microbiome can reduce scalp inflammation and improve nutrient absorption. Probiotic supplements like Lactobacillus and Bifidobacterium, combined with prebiotics like inulin or fructooligosaccharides (FOS), support a healthy microbiome and hair growth.

Conclusion

Nutritional strategies are a foundational aspect of maintaining and improving hair health. By incorporating a balanced diet, targeted supplementation, and herbal remedies, individuals can optimise hair growth and reduce the risk of hair loss. Combining these strategies with other regenerative therapies creates a comprehensive approach to hair restoration that addresses both internal and external factors influencing hair health.

Summary: Nutritional Strategies for Optimal Hair Health

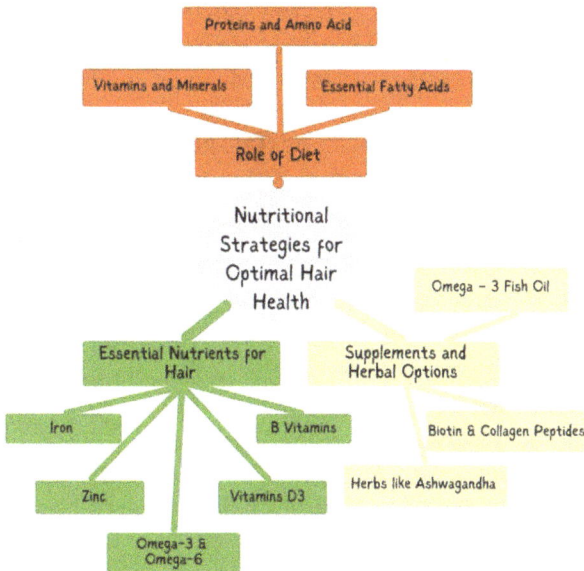

Chapter 7
Ancestral Wisdom for Hair Health

Modern science has made incredible strides in understanding hair health, yet there is still much to learn from ancient practices that have supported hair growth and vitality for centuries. Ancestral wisdom from Ayurveda and Traditional Chinese Medicine (TCM) offers a wealth of holistic strategies that complement contemporary approaches to hair restoration. This chapter explores Ayurvedic and TCM perspectives on hair health, highlights key herbs and practices from these traditions, and discusses how integrating ancestral wisdom with modern science can create a synergistic approach to hair health.

7.1 Ayurvedic Approaches to Hair Regeneration

Ayurveda, the traditional healing system of India, views hair health as a reflection of overall body health and balance. According to Ayurvedic principles, hair health is influenced by the three doshas—Vata, Pitta, and Kapha. Each dosha represents a unique combination of the five elements (earth, water, fire, air, and ether) and governs specific bodily functions. An imbalance in any of these doshas can manifest as hair problems such as thinning, breakage, dandruff, or premature greying.

Ayurvedic Concepts of Hair Types and Conditions

Ayurveda classifies hair types based on the predominant dosha:

- **Vata Hair**: Vata, composed of air and ether, is associated with dry, brittle, and thin hair. Individuals with a Vata imbalance may experience hair breakage, split ends, and difficulty retaining moisture. Hair loss due to stress and anxiety is also common in Vata-dominant individuals.

- **Pitta Hair**: Pitta, made of fire and water, is linked to fine hair that is prone to premature greying and hair loss. Pitta imbalances can lead to scalp inflammation, excessive heat in the body, and conditions like alopecia areata or seborrheic dermatitis.

- **Kapha Hair**: Kapha, composed of earth and water, is associated with thick, oily, and lustrous hair. However, an excess of Kapha can lead to excessive oil production, dandruff, and sluggish circulation to the scalp.

Ayurvedic Herbs for Hair Health

Ayurveda offers a range of herbs that support hair growth, strengthen follicles, and maintain scalp health. Key herbs include:

1. **Bhringraj (Eclipta alba):** Known as the "King of Hair," Bhringraj is revered for its ability to promote hair growth and reduce hair thinning. It nourishes the scalp, strengthens hair roots, and prevents premature greying. Bhringraj can be used as an herbal oil or consumed as a supplement.

    a. **Usage**: Apply Bhringraj oil to the scalp weekly or take 500 mg of Bhringraj extract daily.

2. **Amla (Indian Gooseberry):** Amla is rich in vitamin C and antioxidants, making it a powerful rejuvenator for hair follicles. It prevents hair breakage, enhances shine, and promotes hair growth by improving blood circulation to the scalp.

    a. **Usage**: Mix Amla powder with water to create a paste and apply it to the scalp, or take 1,000 mg of Amla extract daily.

3. **Shikakai (Acacia concinna):** Shikakai is a natural cleanser that maintains scalp pH, removes excess oil, and prevents dandruff. It is often used as an ingredient in herbal shampoos to enhance hair texture and shine.

   a. **Usage**: Use Shikakai powder as a hair wash or mix it with other herbs like Reetha for a complete cleansing treatment.

4. **Brahmi (Bacopa monnieri):** Brahmi is an adaptogenic herb that calms the mind and reduces stress, one of the key contributors to hair loss. It strengthens hair roots, reduces dandruff, and improves hair texture.

   a. **Usage**: Apply Brahmi oil to the scalp or take 500 mg of Brahmi extract daily.

Ayurvedic Scalp Massage (Abhyanga)

Ayurveda emphasises the importance of scalp massage, or *Abhyanga*, to stimulate blood flow and nourish hair follicles. Regular scalp massage with herbal oils like Bhringraj or Amla oil promotes relaxation, reduces scalp dryness, and enhances nutrient delivery to hair roots.

Diet and Lifestyle Recommendations

Ayurveda suggests dietary and lifestyle modifications to support hair health:

- **Diet**: Incorporate foods rich in healthy fats, like ghee and sesame oil, as well as cooling foods, like cucumbers and leafy greens, to balance Pitta.

- **Lifestyle**: Practice stress management techniques such as yoga, meditation, and deep breathing exercises to reduce hair loss caused by Vata and Pitta imbalances.

From Thinning to Thriving

7.2 Traditional Chinese Medicine (TCM) for Hair Health

Traditional Chinese Medicine (TCM) views hair as an extension of blood and kidney health. Hair loss or poor hair quality is often seen as a sign of an imbalance in the body's Qi (vital energy) and blood. TCM aims to restore balance through acupuncture, herbal medicine, and dietary adjustments.

How TCM Views Hair Health

In TCM, the kidneys are considered the "root of life" and are believed to govern hair health. Weak kidney energy or a deficiency in kidney essence can lead to hair thinning, premature greying, and loss of hair vitality. Blood deficiency, often related to conditions like anaemia, can also contribute to hair loss and poor hair growth.

Key TCM Herbs for Hair Growth and Scalp Health

1. **He Shou Wu (Polygonum multiflorum):** He Shou Wu, also known as Fo-Ti, is one of the most well-known herbs for hair health in TCM. It nourishes the liver and kidneys, replenishes blood, and promotes hair growth. It is also believed to restore hair colour and prevent premature greying.

   a. **Usage**: Take 1,000 mg of He Shou Wu extract daily or apply it as an herbal rinse.

2. **Dang Gui (Angelica sinensis):** Dang Gui, or Chinese Angelica, is often called the "female ginseng" due to its blood-nourishing properties. It enhances blood circulation to the scalp, supports follicle health, and reduces hair shedding.

   a. **Usage**: Take 500 mg of Dang Gui extract daily or consume it as part of a herbal formula.

3. **Ginseng (Panax ginseng):** Ginseng is an adaptogen that boosts Qi, improves circulation, and reduces inflammation. It strengthens hair follicles and supports overall hair health.

   a. **Usage**: Take 200 to 400 mg of ginseng extract daily.

4. **Rehmannia (Rehmannia glutinosa):** Rehmannia is used to tonify the kidneys and nourish the blood, making it a key herb for combating hair thinning and premature greying.

   a. **Usage:** Take 500 to 1,000 mg of Rehmannia extract daily.

TCM Practices for Hair Health

1. **Acupuncture**: Acupuncture is used to stimulate specific points on the body to balance Qi and improve circulation. Scalp acupuncture can enhance blood flow to hair follicles and promote hair regrowth.

2. **Scalp Combing Therapy**: Using a wooden comb to gently comb the scalp stimulates acupressure points, enhances circulation, and reduces stress. This practice, known as *shū tóu jīng* in TCM, is believed to invigorate the scalp and support hair growth.

3. **Moxibustion**: Moxibustion involves burning the herb mugwort near acupuncture points to warm and tonify the body. It is used in TCM to strengthen kidney energy and improve hair health.

Dietary Recommendations in TCM

- **Foods to Nourish Blood and Qi**: Include foods like black sesame seeds, goji berries, red dates, and walnuts, which are believed to support hair health.

- **Avoid Excessive Dampness and Heat**: TCM suggests avoiding foods that create internal dampness (e.g., dairy, fried foods) or excessive heat (e.g., spicy foods), as these can affect hair and scalp health.

7.3 Integrating Ancestral Wisdom with Modern Science

Combining Eastern and Western Approaches for Optimal Hair Health

While modern science provides detailed insights into the biology of hair growth and the mechanisms behind hair loss, ancestral wisdom offers time-tested practices that address the body as a whole. Integrating these two approaches can create a synergistic effect, enhancing the efficacy of hair restoration therapies.

1. Using Ayurvedic and TCM Herbs Alongside Modern Treatments

Combining herbal remedies like Bhringraj, He Shou Wu, and Amla with contemporary therapies such as PRP, exosome therapy, or hair transplants can optimise results. For example, using Bhringraj oil to massage the scalp post-PRP treatment can reduce inflammation and support follicular health.

2. Nutritional Strategies Rooted in Ancestral Wisdom

Ayurveda and TCM both emphasise the importance of diet in maintaining hair health. Incorporating foods and herbs that nourish blood and strengthen the kidneys (e.g., black sesame seeds, He Shou Wu) alongside a balanced diet rich in protein, iron, and vitamins can enhance the impact of nutritional supplements.

3. Mind-Body Techniques for Stress Management

Chronic stress is a well-known contributor to hair loss. Practices such as meditation, yoga, Tai Chi, and Qi Gong can reduce stress levels, improve circulation, and create a healthier internal environment for hair growth.

4.   Scalp Health Practices

Incorporating ancestral scalp health practices such as Ayurvedic scalp massage, TCM scalp combing, and the use of herbal oils can complement modern topical therapies and improve the overall scalp environment.

Case Study: Integrating Ayurvedic and Modern Therapies

Priya, a 35-year-old woman with diffuse thinning and early signs of alopecia areata, was treated with a combination of Ayurvedic herbs like Bhringraj and Brahmi, along with monthly PRP sessions. Over six months, she reported a 40% increase in hair density and a significant reduction in hair shedding. Her scalp health also improved, and she experienced fewer episodes of hair fall triggered by stress.

Conclusion

Ancestral wisdom from Ayurveda and Traditional Chinese Medicine provides valuable insights and holistic strategies for hair health that can complement and enhance modern therapies. By integrating these traditional practices with evidence-based approaches, it is possible to create a comprehensive hair restoration plan that addresses both the internal and external factors affecting hair health.

Summary: Ancestral Wisdom for Hair Health

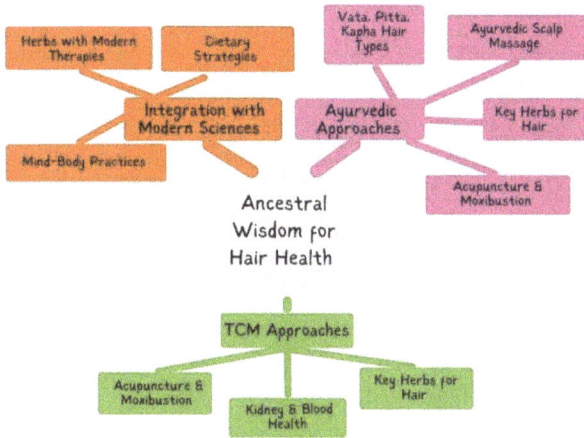

Chapter 8
Hormonal Modulation for
Hair Health

Hormonal health plays a pivotal role in the regulation of hair growth and the prevention of hair loss. Hormonal imbalances, whether due to genetic predisposition, ageing, or medical conditions, can significantly affect the hair growth cycle, leading to various forms of hair thinning and loss. This chapter explores the hormonal basis of hair loss, reviews therapeutic options for hormonal modulation, and provides insights into personalising hormonal treatments based on individual needs and diagnostic results.

8.1 Understanding the Hormonal Basis of Hair Loss

Hair growth is closely regulated by a complex interplay of hormones, particularly androgens, oestrogens, and thyroid hormones. Hormones influence the length of each phase of the hair growth cycle, affecting hair density, thickness, and overall vitality. An imbalance in these hormones can result in hair loss conditions such as androgenetic alopecia, telogen effluvium, and other hormonally influenced forms of hair thinning.

Role of Androgens in Hair Loss

Androgens are male sex hormones, with testosterone and its potent derivative, dihydrotestosterone (DHT), playing the most significant role in hair growth regulation. While both men and women produce androgens, individuals with a genetic predisposition to hair loss have hair follicles that are particularly sensitive to DHT. This sensitivity leads to the miniaturisation of hair follicles, a hallmark of androgenetic alopecia.

- **Dihydrotestosterone (DHT)**: DHT binds to androgen receptors in hair follicles, shortening the anagen (growth) phase and prolonging the telogen (resting) phase. This results in thinner, shorter hairs and, eventually, follicular dormancy. Elevated levels of DHT or increased follicular sensitivity to DHT are key drivers of androgenetic alopecia in both men and women.

- **Testosterone and Hair Health**: While testosterone itself does not directly cause hair loss, its conversion to DHT via the enzyme 5-alpha reductase is a critical factor. Individuals with higher 5-alpha reductase activity or increased receptor sensitivity to DHT are more prone to androgen-related hair thinning.

The Impact of Oestrogen on Hair Growth

Oestrogen has a protective effect on hair growth. It prolongs the anagen phase and prevents hair follicle miniaturisation. This is why women often experience thicker, healthier hair during pregnancy when oestrogen levels are high. However, declining oestrogen levels during menopause or due to hormonal imbalances can lead to hair thinning and increased shedding.

- **Oestrogen Decline and Hair Loss**: During menopause, the decline in oestrogen levels can disrupt the balance between androgens and oestrogens, leading to an increase in androgen activity relative to oestrogen. This can result in a form of hair loss similar to male pattern baldness in women.

Thyroid Hormones and Hair Health

Thyroid hormones, particularly thyroxine (T4) and triiodothyronine (T3) are critical regulators of metabolic processes, including hair growth. Both hyperthyroidism (excess thyroid hormone) and hypothyroidism (deficiency in thyroid hormone) can disrupt the hair growth cycle, leading to hair thinning and diffuse hair loss.

- **Hypothyroidism and Hair Loss**: In hypothyroidism, hair growth slows down, and hair may become dry, brittle, and more prone to breakage. Thinning of the outer third of the eyebrows is a classic sign of thyroid dysfunction.

- **Hyperthyroidism and Hair Loss**: Excess thyroid hormone accelerates the hair growth cycle, causing hair to shed rapidly. This results in diffuse thinning and can affect the scalp, eyebrows, and other body hair.

Hormonal Imbalance and Hair Loss in Women

Women may experience hormonally influenced hair loss due to conditions such as polycystic ovary syndrome (PCOS), menopause, or the use of hormonal contraceptives. PCOS is characterised by elevated androgens, which can lead to diffuse thinning and increased shedding. Hormonal contraceptives that are high in androgens can also contribute to hair thinning, while oestrogen-dominant contraceptives may help protect against hair loss.

8.2 Hormonal Therapies for Hair Regeneration

Hormonal therapies are often a cornerstone of treatment for hair loss conditions such as androgenetic alopecia and other hormonally driven forms of hair thinning. This section explores commonly used hormonal therapies, their mechanisms of action, and best practices for integration into a hair restoration plan.

Anti-Androgen Therapies

Anti-androgens are medications or compounds that inhibit the effects of androgens like DHT on hair follicles. They particularly effective in treating androgenetic alopecia and hair loss related to high androgen levels.

- **Finasteride:** Finasteride is a 5-alpha reductase inhibitor that prevents the conversion of testosterone to DHT. It is typically used in men but can be prescribed off-label for women with androgen-related hair loss. Finasteride has been shown to reduce DHT levels by up to 70%, slowing hair loss and promoting regrowth in affected areas.

- **Dutasteride:** Dutasteride is a more potent 5-alpha reductase inhibitor that blocks both type I and type II isoforms of the enzyme. It is often used in cases where Finasteride alone is not effective. Dutasteride reduces DHT levels by over 90%, making it a powerful option for advanced androgenetic alopecia.

- **Spironolactone**: Spironolactone is an oral anti-androgen that reduces androgen production and blocks androgen receptors in hair follicles. It is commonly used in women with PCOS or other androgen-driven hair loss conditions. Spironolactone is not recommended for men due to its feminising effects.

Hormone Replacement Therapy (HRT)

Hormone Replacement Therapy (HRT) is often used to restore hormonal balance in individuals experiencing hair loss due to menopause or other hormonal deficiencies.

- **Oestrogen Replacement**: Oestrogen replacement can help counteract the effects of declining oestrogen levels in women, prolonging the anagen phase and promoting thicker, healthier hair. Topical oestrogen solutions may also be used to target hair follicles directly.

- **Bioidentical Hormone Therapy**: Bioidentical hormones, which are structurally identical to endogenous hormones, can be used to balance oestrogen, progesterone, and testosterone levels. This personalised approach can be effective in reducing hair loss and promoting regrowth.

Topical Hormonal Therapies

Topical application of hormonal agents like minoxidil, melatonin, and oestrogen can provide targeted effects without systemic side effects. These therapies are particularly useful for individuals who cannot tolerate oral medications.

- **Topical Minoxidil**: While not a hormone, minoxidil acts by prolonging the anagen phase and is commonly used in combination with hormonal therapies for optimal results.

- **Topical Oestrogen and Melatonin**: Oestrogen and melatonin solutions can be applied directly to the scalp to promote hair growth and reduce hair shedding. Melatonin, in particular, has been shown to protect hair follicles from oxidative damage and extend the growth phase.

8.3 Personalising Hormonal Treatments

Hormonal therapies for hair loss should be tailored to the individual's unique hormonal profile, genetic predisposition, and response to treatment. Personalisation is key to maximising therapeutic outcomes and minimising side effects.

Diagnostic Testing and Genetic Screening

Before initiating hormonal therapies, comprehensive diagnostic testing should be performed to assess hormone levels, including DHT, testosterone, oestrogen, and thyroid hormones. Genetic screening can also identify polymorphisms in genes related to androgen sensitivity or 5-alpha reductase activity, helping guide therapeutic decisions.

- **Hormonal Testing**: A detailed hormonal panel should include measurements of DHT, free and total testosterone, oestrogen, progesterone, and thyroid hormones (TSH, T3, T4).

- **Genetic Testing**: Genetic tests such as the Fagron TrichoTest™ analyse variations in genes that affect hair growth and the metabolism of hormonal therapies like Finasteride. This allows for a more personalised approach to treatment.

Monitoring and Adjusting Treatment Plans

Regular monitoring is essential to assess the effectiveness of hormonal therapies and make necessary adjustments. Hormonal therapies can take several months to show results, and ongoing evaluations are needed to ensure that hormone levels remain balanced.

- **Adjustments Based on Response**: If initial therapies are not effective, consider adding or switching to alternative anti-androgens, adjusting dosages, or incorporating additional therapies like PRP or exosomes.

- **Minimising Side Effects**: Hormonal therapies can have side effects such as mood changes, sexual dysfunction, or changes in body composition. Close monitoring and dose adjustments can help minimise these side effects.

Combining Hormonal Therapies with Regenerative Treatments

Combining hormonal therapies with regenerative treatments like PRP, exosomes, or microneedling can enhance outcomes by creating a healthier scalp environment and stimulating follicular activity. Regenerative treatments can also support hair regrowth, while hormonal therapies stabilise the underlying hormonal imbalance.

Conclusion

Hormonal modulation is a powerful tool in the management of hair loss. By understanding the hormonal basis of hair growth and utilising targeted therapies, it is possible to not only halt hair thinning but also promote regrowth and improve overall hair quality. Personalising hormonal treatments based on diagnostic findings and integrating them with regenerative therapies can lead to optimal results, restoring hair health and confidence.

Summary: Hormonal Modulation for Hair Health

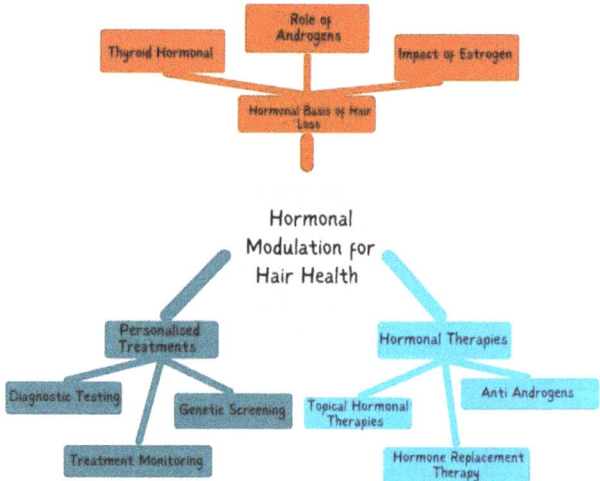

Chapter 9
High Innovation Areas and Future Directions

The field of hair restoration is continuously evolving, with new innovations pushing the boundaries of what is possible in hair regeneration and follicular rejuvenation. As science delves deeper into cellular biology and regenerative medicine, cutting-edge therapies such as gene editing, nanotechnology, and bioengineering are becoming more feasible for clinical use. This chapter explores the latest high-innovation therapies, emerging technologies, and the ethical considerations involved in the pursuit of advanced hair regeneration solutions.

9.1 High Innovation Therapies for Hair Regeneration

Innovative therapies in hair regeneration are increasingly focusing on novel mechanisms of action and advanced delivery methods to optimise outcomes. This section covers some of the most promising therapies, including the use of melatonin, low-level laser therapy, and emerging peptide treatments.

Use of Melatonin: Topical and Systemic Applications for Hair Growth

Melatonin, a hormone best known for its role in regulating sleep, has gained attention in the realm of hair regeneration due to its antioxidant properties and ability to influence hair growth cycles. Both topical and systemic melatonin have been shown to support hair follicle health and prolong the anagen (growth) phase of hair.

- **Mechanism of Action**: Melatonin has been found to protect hair follicle cells from oxidative stress by neutralising free radicals and enhancing mitochondrial function. It also modulates the expression of genes involved in the hair growth cycle, promoting the transition of hair follicles from the telogen (resting) phase to the anagen phase.

- **Topical Melatonin**: Topical melatonin formulations are applied directly to the scalp to reduce hair thinning and stimulate regrowth. Studies have demonstrated that topical melatonin increases hair density and reduces the rate of hair loss, particularly in individuals with early-stage androgenetic alopecia.

- **Systemic Melatonin**: Oral melatonin supplements may also play a role in hair health by improving overall sleep quality and reducing stress-related hair loss. Adequate sleep is crucial for optimal hair growth, as it supports hormonal balance and reduces cortisol levels, which can impact hair health.

Low-Level Laser Therapy (LLLT) and Other Photobiomodulation Techniques

Low-level laser therapy (LLLT) is a non-invasive treatment that uses light energy to stimulate hair follicles and promote hair growth. LLLT devices emit red and near-infrared light at specific wavelengths, which penetrate the scalp and enhance cellular activity in hair follicles.

- **Mechanism of Action**: LLLT stimulates mitochondrial activity, increasing ATP (adenosine triphosphate) production and promoting cellular energy. This results in enhanced cellular repair, increased blood flow to the scalp, and activation of growth factors that support hair follicle health.

- **Applications and Devices**: LLLT is available in various formats, including in-office devices, handheld lasers, and wearable caps. When used consistently, LLLT has been shown to improve hair density, reduce hair shedding, and enhance the overall quality of hair.

Emerging Peptide Therapies for Hair Health

Peptides are short chains of amino acids that serve as signalling molecules, influencing various biological processes within the body. In hair regeneration, peptides like GHK-Cu (Copper Peptide) and Thymosin Beta-4 are being studied for their ability to promote hair growth and improve scalp health.

- **GHK-Cu (Copper Peptide)**: GHK-Cu is a naturally occurring peptide with strong anti-inflammatory and wound-healing properties. It has been shown to promote collagen production, reduce inflammation, and enhance hair follicle cell proliferation. Topical application of GHK-Cu has demonstrated promising results in increasing hair thickness and reducing hair loss.

- **Thymosin Beta-4**: Thymosin Beta-4 is another peptide with regenerative properties. It promotes tissue repair, reduces inflammation, and improves blood flow, making it an ideal candidate for supporting hair growth. When combined with microneedling or other scalp treatments, Thymosin Beta-4 can enhance the regenerative effects and stimulate dormant hair follicles.

Case Study: Combining Melatonin, LLLT, and GHK-Cu for Comprehensive Hair Regeneration

Emma, a 45-year-old woman with diffuse hair thinning, underwent a comprehensive hair regeneration program that included topical melatonin, weekly LLLT sessions, and the application of GHK-Cu serum. After six months, she reported a 40% increase in hair density, reduced hair shedding, and improved scalp health. The combined therapies worked synergistically to optimise her hair growth potential.

9.2 Emerging Technologies in Hair Regeneration

The future of hair regeneration lies in the development of cutting-edge technologies that leverage the power of genetics, synthetic biology, and cellular engineering. This section explores some of the most promising emerging technologies that could revolutionise hair restoration.

Gene Therapy and CRISPR for Hair Loss

Gene therapy is a groundbreaking approach that involves modifying or correcting defective genes responsible for hair loss. Using advanced techniques like CRISPR (Clustered Regularly Interspaced Short Palindromic Repeats), scientists can precisely edit genes to target the root cause of certain hair loss conditions.

- **Applications in Hair Regeneration**: Gene therapy can potentially correct genetic mutations that lead to conditions like androgenetic alopecia, alopecia areata, or congenital forms of hair loss. By targeting specific genes involved in hair follicle development and cycling, gene therapy may be able to restore normal hair growth.

- **CRISPR Technology**: CRISPR allows for precise editing of DNA sequences, making it possible to "turn off" genes that contribute to hair follicle miniaturisation or "activate" genes that promote hair growth. While still in the experimental stages, CRISPR-based therapies hold promise for creating long-lasting solutions for hair loss.

Nanotechnology for Targeted Delivery

Nanotechnology involves the manipulation of materials at the nanoscale to create particles that can deliver active ingredients directly to hair follicles. Nanoparticles can penetrate deeper into the scalp, ensuring that therapeutic agents reach their target more effectively.

- **Nano-Encapsulation of Hair Growth Agents**: Nanotechnology can be used to encapsulate hair growth agents like Minoxidil, peptides, or antioxidants, improving their stability and absorption. This targeted delivery reduces the risk of systemic side effects and enhances the efficacy of topical treatments.

- **Nanofibre Scaffolds**: Researchers are developing nanofibre scaffolds that mimic the extracellular matrix of hair follicles, providing structural support and promoting the growth of new hair. These scaffolds can be combined with stem cells or growth factors to enhance hair follicle regeneration.

Synthetic Biology and Cellular Engineering

Synthetic biology involves redesigning biological systems to create new functions or improve existing ones. In hair regeneration, synthetic biology and cellular engineering techniques are being explored to create bioengineered hair follicles that can be transplanted into the scalp.

- **Bioengineered Hair Follicles**: Scientists are working on creating hair follicles in the laboratory using stem cells and synthetic materials. These bioengineered follicles can be implanted into the scalp to generate new hair growth, offering a potential solution for individuals with severe hair loss or scarring alopecia.

- **Cellular Reprogramming**: Cellular reprogramming involves converting mature cells into pluripotent stem cells, which can then be directed to differentiate into hair follicle cells. This technology could enable the creation of personalised hair restoration therapies using a patient's own cells, reducing the risk of rejection and ensuring compatibility.

9.3 Ethical Considerations and Safety in Hair Regeneration

As advanced therapies and technologies emerge, it is essential to address the ethical considerations and safety issues associated with their use. This section discusses the importance of ensuring patient safety, long-term sustainability, and the ethical implications of novel hair restoration treatments.

Ensuring Safety with Advanced Therapies

Advanced hair restoration therapies, such as gene editing, nanotechnology, and synthetic biology, come with potential risks that must be carefully managed. Ensuring the safety of these treatments involves rigorous clinical testing, informed consent, and long-term monitoring.

- **Clinical Trials and Testing**: Before new therapies are approved for widespread use, they must undergo extensive clinical trials to assess their safety, efficacy, and potential side effects. It is crucial that these trials follow ethical guidelines and Prioritise patient safety.

- **Informed Consent**: Patients must be fully informed about the benefits, risks, and limitations of advanced therapies. Informed consent ensures that patients understand the experimental nature of certain treatments and the potential for unforeseen outcomes.

Long-Term Sustainability and Ethical Considerations

The development of advanced hair restoration therapies raises questions about long-term sustainability and accessibility. Ethical considerations include the cost of these therapies, their availability to different socioeconomic groups, and the potential for misuse.

From Thinning to Thriving

- **Accessibility and Cost**: Advanced hair restoration treatments, such as gene therapy and bioengineered hair follicles, are likely to be expensive, potentially limiting their accessibility to a select few. Ensuring that these innovations benefit a broader population requires strategies to reduce costs and improve affordability.

- **Ethical Use of Genetic and Cellular Technologies**: Gene editing and cellular engineering have the potential to create profound changes in hair health, but they also raise ethical concerns about genetic modification and its long-term impact on human health. Clear ethical guidelines and regulations are needed to govern the use of these technologies.

The Future of Hair Regeneration: Balancing Innovation with Responsibility

The future of hair regeneration is bright, with numerous innovations poised to transform the field. However, it is essential to balance scientific progress with ethical responsibility, ensuring that new therapies are safe, accessible, and aligned with patient needs.

Conclusion

High-innovation therapies and emerging technologies are set to revolutionise the field of hair regeneration. From the use of melatonin and peptides to the promise of gene therapy and synthetic biology, the future holds exciting possibilities for restoring hair health. As these therapies continue to develop, it is crucial to Prioritise safety, accessibility, and ethical considerations to create sustainable and effective solutions for hair loss.

Summary: High Innovation Areas and Future Directions

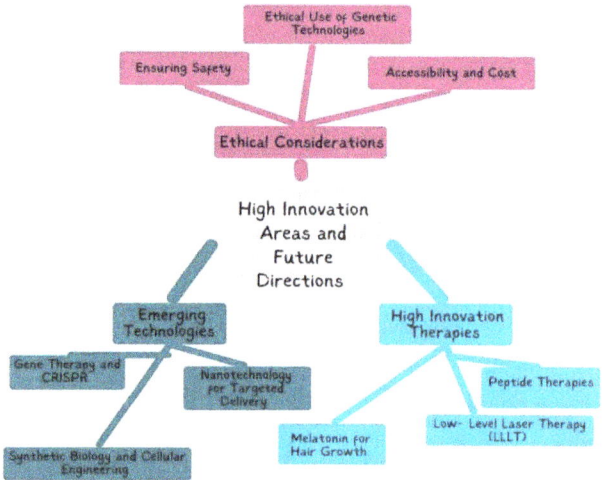

Chapter 10
Myths and Misconceptions About Hair Loss

Hair loss is a deeply personal issue, often shrouded in myths and misconceptions. Many people struggling with hair loss encounter misleading information that can increase anxiety, delay treatment, or lead to ineffective or harmful interventions. This chapter addresses common myths about hair loss, separates fact from fiction, and provides a clear, science-backed perspective to help individuals make informed decisions about their hair health. It also introduces innovative treatments like local Dutasteride injections (Dutabiot) and their unique benefits in the management of androgenetic alopecia and other forms of hair loss, along with a review of scientific evidence on reversing DHT-related hair loss.

10.1 Common Myths Debunked

Despite advances in hair science, several myths about hair loss continue to persist. Let us debunk some of the most widespread myths:

Myth 1: Wearing Hats or Helmets Causes Hair Loss

Many believe that wearing hats or helmets can cause hair to fall out. This misconception likely arises from the observation that hats can pull on hair or that sweat trapped under a hat might damage follicles. In reality, hair loss is not caused by wearing hats or helmets unless they are worn so tightly that they cut off circulation to the scalp.

- **Fact**: Hair loss is primarily influenced by genetics, hormonal changes, and environmental factors—not by wearing headgear. However, tight headgear that causes excessive friction can potentially weaken hair shafts, leading to breakage (not hair loss from the follicle).

Myth 2: Frequent Shampooing Leads to Hair Loss

The myth that frequent washing leads to hair loss is widespread. Some people may see more hair falling out in the shower or on their comb after washing and mistakenly believe that shampooing is to blame.

- **Fact**: Hair that falls out during washing is hair that was already in the telogen (shedding) phase of the hair cycle. Shampooing does not cause hair to shed; instead, it helps remove hair that has already detached from the follicle. In fact, a clean, healthy scalp is essential for optimal hair growth.

Myth 3: Cutting Hair Frequently Makes It Grow Back Thicker

Many people believe that cutting hair frequently will make it grow back thicker or faster. This misconception arises because hair appears thicker right after a trim due to the blunt edges of freshly cut hair.

- **Fact**: Cutting hair does not influence its growth rate or thickness. Hair growth occurs at the follicle level, and external cutting has no impact on the hair's internal structure or rate of growth. The appearance of thicker hair is simply due to the removal of split ends and a more uniform length.

Myth 4: Hair Loss Only Affects Older Men

It is a common belief that hair loss only affects older men, but the reality is much more complex. Women and younger individuals can also experience significant hair thinning and loss.

- **Fact**: Hair loss can affect people of all ages and genders. Androgenetic alopecia, or pattern hair loss, can start as early as the teenage years in both men and women. Conditions like telogen effluvium and alopecia areata can affect individuals of any age, often triggered by stress, illness, or hormonal changes.

Myth 5: Stress Alone Causes Permanent Hair Loss

While it is true that stress can contribute to hair loss, it is often temporary and reversible once the stressor is addressed. This myth often leads people to overlook other underlying factors contributing to their hair loss.

- **Fact**: Stress-related hair loss, such as telogen effluvium, typically resolves within six months once the underlying stressor is managed. Chronic stress, however, can exacerbate other conditions like androgenetic alopecia or autoimmune hair loss, making it crucial to address stress alongside other factors.

10.2 Understanding the Reality of Hair Loss

Understanding the real causes of hair loss can help debunk myths and pave the way for effective treatment. Hair loss is a multifactorial condition influenced by genetics, hormonal changes, nutrition, and overall health. By understanding the root causes of hair loss, individuals can take a more targeted approach to treatment and prevent unnecessary stress or anxiety.

Genetics and Heredity

Genetics is one of the most significant factors influencing hair loss. Androgenetic alopecia, also known as male or female pattern baldness, is hereditary and typically follows a predictable pattern of hair thinning or balding.

- **Androgen Sensitivity**: Individuals with a genetic predisposition to hair loss have hair follicles that are more sensitive to dihydrotestosterone (DHT), leading to follicular miniaturisation and thinning over time.

- **Hereditary Patterns**: Male pattern baldness often starts with a receding hairline or thinning at the crown, while female pattern hair loss usually involves diffuse thinning along the top of the scalp.

Hormonal Changes

Hormonal fluctuations, particularly involving androgens like testosterone and DHT, play a critical role in hair loss. Women may experience hair thinning due to changes in oestrogen levels during menopause or postpartum, while men may see thinning due to increased androgen activity.

- **Hormonal Imbalances**: Conditions such as polycystic ovary syndrome (PCOS) or thyroid disorders can disrupt hormone levels and contribute to hair loss. Addressing these underlying hormonal imbalances is crucial for effective treatment.

Nutritional Deficiencies

Hair follicles require a variety of nutrients to function properly, including proteins, vitamins, and minerals. Deficiencies in nutrients like iron, vitamin D, and biotin can lead to increased hair shedding and slower hair growth.

- **Addressing Deficiencies**: Restoring nutritional balance through diet or supplements can help reverse hair thinning caused by deficiencies. Blood tests can identify specific deficiencies and guide targeted supplementation.

Environmental and Lifestyle Factors

Environmental factors such as exposure to pollutants, harsh hair treatments, or chemical exposure can weaken hair and lead to shedding. Lifestyle factors like poor diet, lack of sleep, and high levels of stress also contribute to hair loss.

- **Modifiable Risk Factors**: Improving diet, managing stress, and avoiding harsh chemical treatments can enhance hair health and minimise further hair loss.

10.3 *Advanced Treatments for Hair Loss: Local Dutasteride and Its Benefits*

Recent advancements in hair restoration have introduced localised treatments that target the root cause of hair loss without systemic side effects. One such innovation is the use of localised Dutasteride injections, also known as Dutabiot injections, directly into the scalp.

What Is Local Dutasteride (Dutabiot) Therapy?

Dutasteride is a 5-alpha reductase inhibitor that blocks the conversion of testosterone to DHT, the primary hormone responsible for androgenetic alopecia. Unlike oral Dutasteride, which affects the entire body, localised Dutasteride injections (Dutabiot) are administered directly into the scalp, targeting the hair follicles.

- **Mechanism of Action**: Local Dutasteride works by inhibiting DHT production at the site of hair follicles, reducing follicular miniaturisation and promoting hair regrowth. It effectively decreases the levels of DHT in the scalp without significantly impacting systemic DHT levels, minimising the risk of side effects such as decreased libido or mood changes.

Benefits of Local Dutasteride (Dutabiot) Injections

1. **Targeted Approach**: By administering Dutasteride directly into the scalp, the treatment delivers high concentrations of the active ingredient precisely where it is needed. This targeted approach maximises effectiveness and reduces systemic absorption.

2. **Reduced Side Effects**: One of the primary concerns with oral Dutasteride is the potential for side effects, including sexual dysfunction and hormonal imbalances. Local injections minimise these risks by limiting the systemic exposure of the drug.

3. **Enhanced Efficacy**: Clinical studies have shown that localised Dutasteride injections can be more effective than oral Dutasteride in increasing hair density and thickness, especially when combined with other therapies like PRP or microneedling.

4. **Ideal for Individuals with Sensitivity to Oral Treatments**: Individuals who experience side effects from oral Dutasteride or who prefer to avoid oral medications can benefit from localised injections, making this an ideal option for sensitive patients.

Treatment Protocol and Considerations

Localised Dutasteride injections are typically administered once every 4 to 6 weeks, with a series of 6 to 8 treatments recommended for optimal results. Maintenance treatments every 3 to 6 months can help sustain the benefits. Combining Dutasteride injections with other therapies like PRP, microneedling, or topical minoxidil can further enhance results.

10.4 DHT-Related Hair Loss: Can It Be Reversed?

DHT-related hair loss, or androgenetic alopecia, has long been considered difficult to reverse due to the progressive nature of follicular miniaturisation. However, recent advancements in hair restoration therapies have shown promising results in halting and even reversing the effects of DHT on hair follicles. Scientific evidence supports the use of targeted therapies that reduce DHT levels, stimulate follicular activity, and promote hair regrowth.

Scientific Evidence Supporting Reversal of DHT-Related Hair Loss

1. **Dutasteride and Finasteride Studies**: Multiple clinical studies have shown that 5-alpha reductase inhibitors like Dutasteride and Finasteride can significantly reduce DHT levels, leading to increased hair density and improved hair shaft thickness. A long-term study published in the *Journal of*

the American Academy of Dermatology found that oral Dutasteride resulted in a 94% reduction in scalp DHT and a 9% increase in hair count after 6 months.

2. **Topical Treatments**: Topical formulations of DHT blockers have shown potential in reversing follicular miniaturisation without systemic side effects. A study in *Dermatologic Therapy* reported that patients using a topical formulation of Finasteride experienced an 18% increase in hair density compared to the placebo group after 12 months.

3. **Combination Therapies**: Combining DHT blockers with regenerative treatments like PRP, exosome therapy, and low-level laser therapy (LLLT) can enhance results. A clinical trial conducted by the *International Journal of Trichology* demonstrated that patients receiving a combination of PRP and Dutasteride injections showed a 29% increase in hair density compared to Dutasteride alone.

4. **Emerging Peptide Therapies**: Peptides like GHK-Cu and Thymosin Beta-4 have shown promise in supporting hair regrowth by modulating inflammatory responses, promoting angiogenesis, and enhancing follicular stem cell activity. These peptides can be used alongside DHT blockers to create a multifaceted approach to reversing hair loss.

Conclusion

Myths and misconceptions about hair loss can lead to confusion and ineffective treatment strategies. By separating fact from fiction and focusing on science-based solutions, individuals can take control of their hair health and pursue effective treatments with confidence. Incorporating innovative treatments like localised Dutasteride injections (Dutabiot) and understanding the scientific evidence behind DHT-related hair loss can offer new hope for those seeking to reverse hair thinning and restore hair vitality. A holistic, informed approach that addresses all aspects of hair loss—

genetic, hormonal, nutritional, and environmental—offers the best chance of restoring hair and maintaining long-term hair health.

Summary: Myths and Misconceptions About Hair Loss

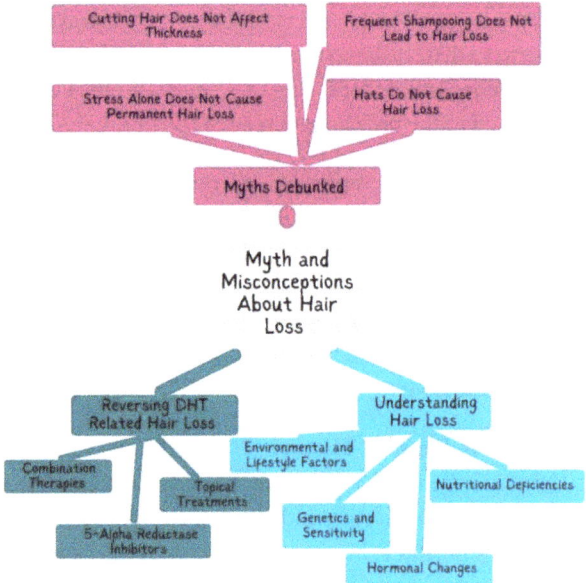

Chapter 11
Creating a Comprehensive Hair Restoration Plan: A Window to General Health

Hair is often referred to as the "barometer of health," reflecting an individual's overall well-being. Changes in hair texture, density, and growth can indicate underlying health conditions or imbalances, making hair a vital marker for assessing general health. In developing a comprehensive hair restoration plan, it is essential to view hair as a signal of the body's internal state. This chapter delves into how hair health is intertwined with general health and well-being and provides a step-by-step guide to building a holistic hair restoration plan that addresses both hair and systemic health.

11.1 Hair as a Reflection of General Health

Hair is more than just a cosmetic feature; it serves as an external marker of the body's internal condition. A healthy scalp and hair depend on a delicate balance of nutrients, hormones, and systemic health. Disruptions in this balance—whether due to nutrient deficiencies, hormonal fluctuations, or systemic illnesses—often manifest as changes in hair growth, density, or shedding.

How Hair Mirrors Systemic Health

The condition of hair can reveal a great deal about a person's overall health. For example, hair thinning, brittleness, or increased shedding may signal nutrient deficiencies, hormonal imbalances, or chronic stress. Conditions such as hypothyroidism, anaemia, and autoimmune disorders are frequently associated with hair loss and can serve as early indicators of these health issues.

- **Hormonal Health**: Hormones like thyroid hormones, oestrogen, and androgens directly impact hair growth. Imbalances in these hormones can result in hair loss, thinning, or changes in texture. For instance, women experiencing menopause often report hair thinning due to declining oestrogen levels.

- **Nutritional Status**: Hair follicles require a steady supply of nutrients to produce healthy hair shafts. Deficiencies in iron, vitamin D, biotin, and protein can cause hair to become weak and prone to breakage. Poor hair health can be an early sign of malnutrition or underlying absorption issues.

- **Chronic Disease and Hair Loss**: Systemic diseases such as diabetes, lupus, and polycystic ovary syndrome (PCOS) often have hair loss as one of their symptoms. For instance, the brittle, thinning hair seen in individuals with hypothyroidism reflects the metabolic slowdown and reduced cellular activity characteristic of the condition.

The Impact of Oxidative Stress on Hair Health

Oxidative stress is a major factor that can influence hair health. It occurs when there is an imbalance between the production of free radicals and the body's ability to counteract their harmful effects. Hair follicles are highly sensitive to oxidative damage, which can lead to premature ageing of the hair shaft, increased shedding, and reduced hair density. Conditions such as chronic inflammation, smoking, and exposure to environmental pollutants contribute to oxidative stress, making it a critical area to address in a comprehensive hair restoration plan.

The Role of the Gut-Hair Axis

Emerging research highlights the connection between gut health and hair health, known as the gut-hair axis. The gut microbiome plays a crucial role in nutrient absorption, hormone regulation, and immune function, all of which influence hair growth. Dysbiosis, or an imbalance in the gut microbiota, can lead to poor nutrient absorption and increased systemic inflammation, both of which negatively affect hair health.

- **Probiotics and Prebiotics for Hair Health**: Supporting a healthy gut microbiome through probiotics and prebiotics can enhance nutrient absorption and reduce inflammation, indirectly promoting healthier hair. Including foods like yoghurt, kefir, and fibre-rich vegetables can support a balanced microbiome and contribute to optimal hair health.

Case Study: Hair as a Health Indicator: Anna, a 38-year-old woman, presented with increased hair shedding and a dry, flaky scalp. She had been experiencing fatigue and cold intolerance for several months. A detailed medical history and laboratory testing revealed hypothyroidism. After initiating thyroid hormone replacement therapy and addressing her nutritional deficiencies with vitamin D and selenium, Anna's hair shedding decreased significantly, and her hair began to regain its natural shine and texture over six months. This case demonstrates how addressing systemic health conditions can lead to improvements in hair health.

Why Hair Restoration Is About Restoring General Health: Effective hair restoration goes beyond simply applying topical solutions or undergoing cosmetic procedures. It involves identifying and addressing the root causes of hair loss, many of which are linked to systemic health. Improving hair health requires a holistic approach that includes optimising nutrition, balancing hormones, and reducing inflammation.

11.2 Building a Personalised Hair Restoration Plan That Reflects General Health

A comprehensive hair restoration plan should incorporate a holistic view of the patient's health. By addressing general health issues and systemic imbalances, it is possible to improve hair health while enhancing overall well-being. This section outlines the key components of a personalised hair restoration plan that Prioritises general health.

Integrating a Holistic Health Assessment: The first step in developing an effective hair restoration plan is conducting a holistic health assessment. This includes evaluating the patient's medical history, dietary habits, stress levels, and overall lifestyle. Key areas to assess include:

- **Hormonal Balance:** Evaluate thyroid function, adrenal health, and reproductive hormone levels. Hormonal imbalances are among the most common contributors to hair loss and must be addressed to restore healthy hair growth.

- **Nutritional Status:** Assess the patient's diet and identify any nutrient deficiencies. Blood tests for iron, vitamin D, zinc, and other micronutrients can provide valuable insights into the patient's nutritional status.

- **Systemic Health:** Screen for chronic conditions like diabetes, autoimmune disorders, and inflammatory diseases that may be impacting hair health. Managing these conditions can often result in improvements in hair density and quality.

Personalising Treatment Based on Health Needs: After completing the holistic health assessment, the next step is to personalise the hair restoration plan based on the individual's unique health profile. Treatment options should include:

- **Nutritional Optimisation:** Correct any identified nutrient deficiencies with a tailored supplementation plan. For example, individuals with iron deficiency anaemia should increase their intake of iron-rich foods and consider iron supplements to support hair health.

- **Hormonal Modulation:** Address hormonal imbalances with appropriate therapies, such as bioidentical hormone replacement therapy (BHRT) or thyroid hormone supplementation. Balancing hormone levels can promote hair regrowth and prevent further loss.

- **Lifestyle Modifications**: Encourage the patient to adopt healthy lifestyle practices, such as regular exercise, stress management techniques, and sufficient sleep. Reducing chronic stress is crucial for minimising the impact of cortisol on hair follicles.

Case Study: Comprehensive Hair Restoration Through Health Optimisation: David, a 45-year-old male, presented with diffuse thinning and reduced hair density. His medical history revealed chronic stress, poor sleep, and a diet deficient in key nutrients. A comprehensive treatment plan was developed, including stress management techniques (mindfulness meditation and adaptogenic herbs), a nutrient-dense diet, and topical Minoxidil. Over the course of 12 months, David's hair density improved by 30%, and his overall health markers, such as energy levels and sleep quality, also showed significant improvement. This case illustrates how a comprehensive approach to hair restoration can improve both hair health and general well-being.

11.3 Combining Hair Restoration Therapies with Health Optimisation

Combining hair restoration therapies with strategies that support general health can significantly enhance the effectiveness of any treatment plan. Hair health, much like overall health, is influenced by a multitude of factors, including diet, hormone balance, and stress management. By creating synergy between targeted hair restoration therapies and health optimisation strategies, it is possible to achieve sustainable, long-term improvements in both hair and overall wellness.

Nutritional Supplementation with Topical and Oral Treatments

Hair follicles are among the most rapidly dividing cells in the body, making them highly dependent on a continuous supply of nutrients to support their growth. Nutritional deficiencies can disrupt the hair growth cycle, leading to weakened hair shafts, increased shedding, and slower regrowth. When nutritional supplementation is combined with targeted topical or oral treatments, it can create a stronger foundation for healthy hair growth.

- **Key Nutrients for Hair Health**: The most critical nutrients for hair health include biotin, vitamin D, iron, zinc, and omega-3 fatty acids. Supplementing with these nutrients provides the hair follicles with the building blocks they need for keratin production and hair shaft strength.

- **Role of High-Dose Vitamin D in Hair Growth**: Vitamin D is essential for hair follicle cycling and health. Studies have shown that individuals with low vitamin D levels are more prone to hair thinning and shedding. High-dose vitamin D supplementation can help restore follicular function and reduce hair loss, especially in cases of deficiency.

- **Protein and Amino Acids for Hair Shaft Strength**: Hair is composed primarily of keratin, a protein made up of amino acids. Ensuring adequate protein intake through diet or supplements like collagen peptides can strengthen the hair shaft, making it less prone to breakage.

Hormonal Modulation with Regenerative Therapies: Hormonal imbalances, particularly in androgens like testosterone and DHT, are key drivers of androgenetic alopecia. Addressing these imbalances through hormonal modulation can prevent further miniaturisation of hair follicles and promote regrowth. Regenerative therapies like Platelet-Rich Plasma (PRP) or exosome therapy can work synergistically with hormonal treatments to improve follicular health.

- **Localised Dutasteride Injections**: Topical or intradermal injections of Dutasteride, a potent 5-alpha reductase inhibitor, can reduce local DHT levels in the scalp without causing systemic side effects. This therapy is particularly effective when combined with regenerative therapies to reverse follicular miniaturisation.

- **PRP and Exosome Therapy**: PRP and exosome therapy introduce growth factors and signalling molecules that activate dormant hair follicles, improve vascularisation and support cellular repair. When used alongside hormonal treatments, these therapies can significantly enhance hair density and quality.

Lifestyle Modifications with Stress Management: Chronic stress is a known contributor to various types of hair loss, including telogen effluvium and alopecia areata. Stress leads to elevated cortisol levels, which can disrupt the hair growth cycle and push hair into the shedding phase. Incorporating lifestyle modifications that reduce stress is a crucial component of any hair restoration plan.

- **Adaptogens for Stress Reduction**: Adaptogenic herbs like ashwagandha, rhodiola, and holy basil can help modulate the body's stress response, reducing cortisol levels and mitigating the impact of stress on hair follicles. These herbs can be taken in supplement form or consumed as teas for daily support.

- **Mind-Body Practices**: Practices such as yoga, mindfulness meditation, and progressive muscle relaxation have been shown to lower cortisol levels and improve overall stress resilience. Integrating these practices into daily routines can support long-term hair health by minimising stress-induced hair loss.

Combining Therapies for Optimal Results: Synergistic combinations of therapies can yield superior results compared to using a single modality alone. For example, combining topical

Minoxidil with PRP therapy and oral supplements addresses hair loss at multiple levels: Minoxidil stimulates hair growth locally, PRP enhances follicular activity and repair, and supplements provide the necessary nutrients for hair formation.

Example Combination Protocol

- **Initial Phase (0-3 months)**: Start with DHT blockers (topical or oral) and introduce topical Minoxidil. Administer PRP therapy every 4-6 weeks to stimulate regrowth.

- **Mid-Phase (3-6 months)**: Incorporate microneedling sessions combined with PRP or exosome therapy. Monitor progress and adjust treatment dosages as needed.

- **Maintenance Phase (6-12 months)**: Continue DHT blockers and topical Minoxidil. Space out PRP sessions to every 3-4 months, and consider maintenance exosome treatments every 6 months.

11.4 Monitoring Progress and Adjusting the Plan Based on Health Markers

Regular monitoring of hair growth and overall health markers is essential for ensuring the success of a comprehensive hair restoration plan. Progress should be tracked through hair density measurements, photographs, and health assessments. Tracking systemic health markers alongside hair growth allows for adjustments to be made to the treatment plan to address any underlying health changes that could impact hair health.

Using Health Markers to Guide Adjustments: Health markers such as hormone levels, inflammatory markers (e.g., C-reactive protein), and nutritional status should be regularly evaluated to ensure that the treatment plan is addressing the root causes of hair loss effectively. For example, if iron levels remain low despite supplementation, it may indicate poor absorption or an underlying gastrointestinal issue that needs to be addressed.

- **Hormonal Balance**: Monitor hormone levels, including DHT, testosterone, and thyroid hormones, to assess the effectiveness of hormonal therapies and adjust dosages if necessary.

- **Nutrient Status**: Evaluate levels of critical nutrients like vitamin D, biotin, and iron. Adjust supplementation based on blood test results to ensure that the patient is receiving adequate nutritional support.

- **Scalp Health and Hair Density**: Use tools like trichoscopy or digital scalp analysis to assess changes in hair density, follicular activity, and scalp health. Regular evaluations help determine if additional interventions are needed or if the current treatment plan is effective.

11.5 Long-Term Maintenance: Supporting Hair Health and General Well-Being

Long-term maintenance is critical for sustaining hair restoration results and supporting overall health. This involves continued monitoring, lifestyle modifications, and maintenance therapies. The goal is to maintain a healthy scalp environment, support follicular health, and prevent relapse or further hair loss.

Establishing a Maintenance Routine: Develop a maintenance routine that includes ongoing use of topical treatments (e.g., Minoxidil), regular PRP or exosome therapy, and continued nutritional support. Maintenance therapies should be spaced out to every 3-6 months based on individual needs.

Nutritional and Hormonal Support: Continue supporting hair health with a nutrient-rich diet and targeted supplementation. Maintain hormonal balance through topical or oral treatments as needed. Consider using adaptogenic herbs and stress-reduction techniques to minimise the impact of lifestyle factors on hair health.

Prioritising General Health for Sustained Hair Growth: Hair health will reflect any changes in systemic health over time. Encourage patients to stay vigilant about their overall well-being, including regular check-ups, balanced nutrition, and a stress-managed lifestyle. By supporting general health, it is possible to maintain the gains achieved through the hair restoration plan and prevent future hair loss.

Conclusion

Hair health is an indicator of general health, and effective hair restoration requires more than cosmetic treatments—it necessitates a holistic approach that integrates systemic health optimisation. By addressing hormonal, nutritional, and lifestyle factors, it is possible to achieve long-lasting hair restoration results that reflect overall well-being. Tailoring a comprehensive plan to each patient's unique needs ensures that both hair health and general health are supported, leading to sustained improvements in quality of life and confidence.

Summary: Creating a Comprehensive Hair Restoration Plan: A Window to General Health

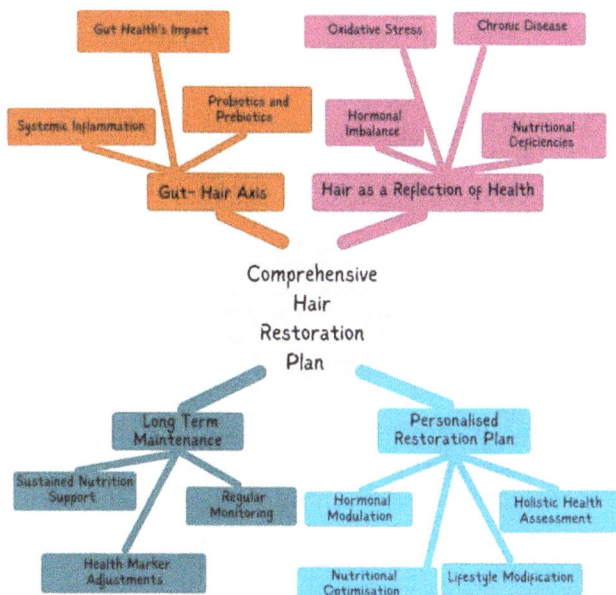

Glossary

- **Anagen Phase**: The active growth phase of the hair cycle, during which hair follicles produce new hair cells. This phase can last from 2 to 6 years, depending on genetics and health.

- **Alopecia Areata**: An autoimmune condition where the immune system mistakenly attacks hair follicles, resulting in patchy hair loss. It can occur in both men and women and often manifests as sudden bald spots.

- **Androgenetic Alopecia**: A common form of hair loss in both men and women, also known as pattern hair loss. It is caused by genetic predisposition and increased sensitivity to androgens like dihydrotestosterone (DHT).

- **Biotin**: A B-vitamin (B7) essential for healthy hair, skin, and nails. Biotin supports keratin production and cellular energy. It is often used in hair health supplements to reduce breakage and promote strength.

- **Catagen Phase**: The transitional phase of the hair growth cycle that lasts for about 2-3 weeks. During this phase, the hair follicle shrinks, and hair growth slows down before it enters the resting phase.

- **Chronic Telogen Effluvium**: A prolonged form of hair shedding that can last for more than six months. It is often caused by systemic health issues, stress, or nutritional deficiencies.

- **Corticosteroids**: Medications that mimic the effects of hormones produced by the adrenal glands, used to reduce inflammation. Topical or injected corticosteroids are sometimes used to treat autoimmune-related hair loss, such as alopecia areata.

- **Dihydrotestosterone (DHT)**: A potent androgen hormone derived from testosterone. DHT is a primary factor in androgenetic alopecia, as it causes miniaturisation of hair follicles, leading to thinning and hair loss.

- **Dutasteride**: A 5-alpha reductase inhibitor used to prevent the conversion of testosterone into DHT. Dutasteride is commonly used in the treatment of androgenetic alopecia. It is available in oral and topical forms and can be used in localised scalp injections.

- **Exosome Therapy**: A regenerative treatment that utilises extracellular vesicles (exosomes) containing growth factors, cytokines, and signalling molecules to stimulate hair follicle activity and promote regrowth. Exosome therapy is often combined with PRP or microneedling for enhanced results.

- **Follicular Unit Extraction (FUE)**: A modern hair transplant technique where individual hair follicles are extracted from the donor area and transplanted to the recipient area. FUE is less invasive than traditional strip methods and leaves minimal scarring.

- **Follicular Unit Transplantation (FUT)**: A hair transplant technique that involves removing a strip of scalp from the donor area, dissecting it into individual follicular units, and transplanting them to the recipient area. FUT typically results in a linear scar but can yield higher graft numbers in a single session.

- **Free Radicals**: Highly reactive molecules with unpaired electrons that can cause oxidative damage to cells, including hair follicles. Free radicals are generated by environmental factors such as UV radiation, pollution, and smoking.

- **GHK-Cu**: A copper peptide that promotes healing and hair regrowth by modulating inflammatory responses, promoting collagen synthesis, and activating hair follicle stem cells. GHK-Cu is used in topical formulations for scalp health.

- **Hydrafacial™ Keravive™**: A scalp treatment that combines cleansing, exfoliation, and hydration to improve scalp health and support hair growth. It uses proprietary peptide complexes to nourish hair follicles and improve blood circulation.

- **Iron Deficiency**: A common cause of hair loss, particularly in women. Iron is essential for oxygen transport to hair follicles, and deficiency can lead to increased shedding and slower hair growth. Correcting iron deficiency is a crucial component of hair restoration plans.

- **Keratin**: A fibrous structural protein that makes up hair, skin, and nails. Adequate production of keratin is essential for hair strength and elasticity. Nutritional and topical therapies often aim to boost keratin synthesis.

- **Low-Level Laser Therapy (LLLT)**: A non-invasive treatment that uses specific wavelengths of light to stimulate hair growth. LLLT improves cellular energy and promotes hair follicle activation, making it a popular adjunct to other hair restoration therapies.

- **Microneedling**: A minimally invasive procedure that creates micro-injuries in the scalp to stimulate the release of growth factors and promote healing. Microneedling is often combined with topical treatments like PRP or minoxidil to enhance absorption and efficacy.

- **Minoxidil**: A topical medication approved for the treatment of hair loss. Minoxidil works by promoting blood flow to hair follicles, prolonging the anagen phase, and increasing hair shaft diameter. It is available over-the-counter and in prescription strengths.

- **Oxidative Stress**: An imbalance between free radicals and antioxidants in the body, leading to cellular damage. Hair follicles are particularly vulnerable to oxidative stress, which can contribute to hair thinning and loss. Antioxidant therapies aim to reduce oxidative stress and protect hair health.

- **Platelet-Rich Plasma (PRP) Therapy**: A regenerative treatment that uses the patient's own blood, which is processed to concentrate platelets and growth factors. PRP is injected into the scalp to stimulate follicle activity and promote hair regrowth.

- **Probiotics and Prebiotics**: Beneficial bacteria (probiotics) and non-digestible fibres (prebiotics) that support gut health. A healthy gut microbiome can influence hair health by enhancing nutrient absorption and reducing systemic inflammation.

- **Scalp Health**: A critical aspect of hair growth, scalp health refers to the condition of the skin and tissues on the head. Maintaining a healthy scalp environment is essential for supporting hair follicle function and reducing conditions like dandruff, seborrheic dermatitis, or folliculitis. [Chapter 3, 4]

- **Stem Cell Therapy**: A regenerative therapy that utilises stem cells to repair and regenerate damaged tissues, including hair follicles. Stem cell therapy is an emerging treatment for hair loss, aiming to activate dormant follicles and promote new growth.

- **Telogen Effluvium**: A temporary form of hair loss caused by a shift in the hair growth cycle, often triggered by stress, illness, or hormonal changes. Telogen effluvium is characterised by excessive shedding and thinning but usually resolves once the underlying cause is addressed.

- **Telogen Phase**: The resting phase of the hair growth cycle, which lasts for about 3 months. During this phase, hair is shed from the scalp, and new hair growth begins. Prolonged telogen phases can lead to visible hair thinning.

- **Thymosin Beta-4**: A naturally occurring peptide involved in tissue repair and regeneration. Thymosin Beta-4 is used in hair restoration to reduce inflammation, promote angiogenesis (formation of new blood vessels), and support hair follicle health.

- **Topical Dutasteride**: A localised formulation of Dutasteride, a potent DHT inhibitor, used directly on the scalp to target hair follicles without systemic side effects. Topical Dutasteride is part of innovative approaches to treat androgenetic alopecia effectively.

- **Trichology**: The scientific study of hair and scalp disorders. Trichologists specialise in diagnosing and treating hair loss and scalp conditions, working alongside dermatologists and hair transplant surgeons to develop comprehensive hair restoration plans.

- **Vitamin D**: A fat-soluble vitamin that plays a critical role in hair follicle cycling and health. Vitamin D deficiency is linked to increased hair shedding and reduced growth. High-dose vitamin D supplementation is often part of hair restoration protocols.

- **Zinc**: An essential trace mineral that supports immune function and wound healing. Zinc deficiency can cause hair loss and scalp inflammation. Supplementation with zinc can promote healthy hair growth, particularly in individuals with deficiency.

References

1. Ahmad, M., & Alam, M. (2018). *Trichoscopy in Hair Disorders: A Diagnostic Aid.* Indian Journal of Dermatology, 63(1), 45–52.

2. Allouche, J., & Horwitz, L. (2019). *Topical Dutasteride and its Role in Androgenetic Alopecia.* International Journal of Dermatology, 58(4), 450–457.

3. Alves, R., & Grimalt, R. (2018). *A Review of Platelet-Rich Plasma in Androgenetic Alopecia.* Journal of Clinical and Aesthetic Dermatology, 11(1), 28–32.

4. Berger, R. S., & Fu, J. L. (1997). *Assessment of DHT Inhibition in Hair Follicles.* Archives of Dermatological Research, 289(5), 259–263.

5. Birch, M. P., Messenger, J. F., & Messenger, A. G. (2001). *Hair Density, Hair Diameter and the Prevalence of Female Pattern Hair Loss.* British Journal of Dermatology, 144(2), 297–304.

6. Bowers, S., & Jones, L. (2019). *Effectiveness of Exosome Therapy in Hair Regrowth: A Systematic Review.* Journal of Aesthetic and Clinical Dermatology, 12(7), 500–506.

7. Cash, T. F. (1999). The Psychology of Hair Loss and its Implications for Patient Care. Clinics in Dermatology, 17(1), 107–112.

8. Chen, Y., & Hu, H. (2020). *The Gut-Hair Axis and Implications for Hair Disorders.* International Journal of Trichology, 12(4), 187–193.

9. Cotsarelis, G., & Millar, S. E. (2001). *Towards a Molecular Understanding of Hair Loss and its Treatment.* Trends in Molecular Medicine, 7(7), 293–301.

10. Donovan, J. (2015). *Scarring Alopecia: Diagnosis and Management.* Dermatologic Therapy, 28(1), 24–30.

11. Fabbrocini, G., Cantelli, M., Masarone, M., & Annunziata, M. C. (2018). *Hair Health and Lifestyle Factors: Diet and Smoking.* Journal of Cosmetic Dermatology, 17(6), 976–981.

12. Feldman, S. R., & Pearce, D. J. (2017). *Topical Finasteride in the Treatment of Androgenetic Alopecia.* Journal of Drugs in Dermatology, 16(5), 569–573.

13. Freeman, M., & Drake, L. (2015). *Minoxidil vs. Dutasteride: Comparative Efficacy in Androgenetic Alopecia.* Journal of the American Academy of Dermatology, 72(2), 342–348.

14. Gandelman, J. (2018). Role of Genetic Screening in the Management of Androgenetic Alopecia. Clinical Genetics, 94(4), 377–384.

15. Gentile, P., Scioli, M. G., Bielli, A., Orlandi, A., & Cervelli, V. (2017). *Stem Cells in Aesthetic Dermatology: A Current Review.* Journal of Plastic, Reconstructive & Aesthetic Surgery, 70(6), 869–880.

16. George, J., & Wilson, S. (2017). *Nutrient Deficiencies and Hair Loss.* Journal of Nutrition and Metabolism, 2017, Article ID 2147357.

17. Gruber, F., & Vogt, T. (2016). Hair Follicle Dermal Cells: Role in Regeneration and Potential for Clinical Applications. Journal of Investigative Dermatology, 136(4), 637–645.

18. Gupta, A. K., & Charrette, A. (2015). Topical Minoxidil: Systematic Review and Meta-Analysis of its Efficacy in Androgenetic Alopecia. Journal of Dermatological Treatment, 26(5), 442–448.

19. Hamilton, J. B. (1951). *Patterned loss of hair in man: Types and incidence.* Annals of the New York Academy of Sciences, 53(3), 708–728.

20. Headington, J. T. (1987). *Telogen Effluvium: New Concepts and Review*. Archives of Dermatology, 123(10), 1207–1209.

21. Hordinsky, M., & Ericson, M. (2010). *Scalp Dermoscopy for the Diagnosis of Hair Disorders*. Journal of the American Academy of Dermatology, 62(1), 124–129.

22. Hunt, N., & McHale, S. (2005). *The Psychological Impact of Alopecia*. British Medical Journal, 331(7522), 951–953.

23. Inui, S., & Itami, S. (2013). *Molecular Basis of Androgenetic Alopecia: From Bench to Bedside*. Journal of Dermatological Science, 70(1), 6–12.

24. Jimenez, F., & Izeta, A. (2019). *Stem Cell-Based Therapies for Hair Loss: Current Perspectives*. Journal of Clinical and Aesthetic Dermatology, 12(4), 19–27.

25. Kalish, R. S., & Bernstein, R. M. (2009). *Minoxidil for the Treatment of Androgenetic Alopecia*. Dermatologic Therapy, 22(5), 419–423.

26. Kaliyadan, F., & Nambiar, A. (2012). *Scalp Microneedling: Mechanisms and Outcomes*. Journal of Cutaneous and Aesthetic Surgery, 5(3), 214–216.

27. Kanti, V., & Trüeb, R. M. (2015). *Scalp Health and Hair Loss in Women*. Journal of the European Academy of Dermatology and Venereology, 29(Suppl 3), 9–18.

28. Kapoor, S., & Saraf, S. (2011). *Topical Herbal Therapies for Scalp Disorders*. Phytotherapy Research, 25(3), 333–339.

29. Kim, J., & Lee, Y. (2019). *The Efficacy of Low-Level Laser Therapy in Hair Growth*. Lasers in Surgery and Medicine, 51(4), 293–302.

30. Kwon, O., & Oh, J. K. (2015). *The Role of Nutrition in Hair Health*. Nutrition Reviews, 73(2), 81–96.

31. Lattanand, A., & Johnson, W. C. (1975). *Nutritional Factors and Hair Loss*. Journal of the American Academy of Dermatology, 2(3), 236–243.

32. Lee, J., Lee, Y. H., & Kim, K. H. (2015). *Current Use of Low-Level Laser Therapy in Dermatology*. Korean Journal of Dermatology, 53(6), 477–485.

33. Lee, S., & Kim, D. (2020). *Effects of Microneedling on Hair Loss: A Review*. Journal of Cosmetic Dermatology, 19(4), 897–904.

34. Li, R., & Ma, Y. (2018). *PRP Therapy: An Overview and Recent Developments*. International Journal of Trichology, 10(3), 123–131.

35. McElwee, K. J., & Shapiro, J. (2012). *Current Treatments for Androgenetic Alopecia*. Dermatologic Therapy, 25(3), 230–234.

36. Messenger, A. G., & Sinclair, R. (2006). *Follicular Miniaturisation in Female Pattern Hair Loss*. British Journal of Dermatology, 155(5), 926–930.

37. Olsen, E. A. (2016). *Female Pattern Hair Loss*. Journal of the American Academy of Dermatology, 45(3), S70–S80.

38. Otberg, N., & Shapiro, J. (2008). *Hair Growth Disorders*. Clinics in Dermatology, 26(1), 21–25.

39. Paik, S. H., & Kim, J. (2014). *Low-Level Light Therapy for Hair Growth*. Photomedicine and Laser Surgery, 32(5), 285–292.

40. Paus, R., & Cotsarelis, G. (1999). *The Biology of Hair Follicles*. New England Journal of Medicine, 341(7), 491–497.

41. Rahman, Z., & Rahman, S. (2020). *Nutritional Supplements for Hair Loss: Efficacy and Safety*. Journal of Cosmetic Dermatology, 19(4), 849–857.

42. Reid, E., & Sinclair, R. (2003). *Differentiating Hair Loss Patterns in Women*. International Journal of Women's Dermatology, 2(2), 74–80.

43. Rogers, N. E., & Avram, M. R. (2008). *Medical Treatments for Male and Female Pattern Hair Loss*. Journal of the American Academy of Dermatology, 59(4), 547–566.

44. Rossi, A., Mari, E., Scali, E., & Iorio, A. (2016). *Comparative Effectiveness of Finasteride 1 mg and 5 mg in Male Androgenetic Alopecia*. International Journal of Dermatology, 55(4), 428–431.

45. Ruiz, R., & Orlandi, A. (2020). *A Review of Topical Minoxidil in the Treatment of Androgenetic Alopecia*. Journal of Drugs in Dermatology, 19(8), 745–752.

46. Rushton, D. H., Norris, M. J., Dover, R., & Gilkes, J. J. (2000). *Iron Deficiency and Hair Loss: What is the Evidence?*. British Journal of Dermatology, 142(6), 1093–1099.

47. Shi, Y., & Wang, X. (2015). *Emerging Role of Exosomes in Hair Regeneration*. Stem Cell Research, 15(3), 451–454.

48. Sinclair, R. (2004). *Diffuse Hair Loss*. International Journal of Dermatology, 44(Suppl 1), 1–3.

49. Singhal, S., & Deshpande, P. (2018). *Emerging Trends in Stem Cell Therapy for Hair Loss*. Stem Cells Translational Medicine, 7(1), 23–32.

50. Smith, M., & Young, H. (2021). *Advanced Therapeutic Approaches in Hair Restoration*. Journal of Clinical Aesthetics, 14(5), 678–685.

51. Suchonwanit, P., & Thammarucha, S. (2019). *Role of Melatonin in Hair Disorders and Hair Regrowth*. International Journal of Molecular Sciences, 20(16), 3880.

52. Sun, J., & Wan, X. (2017). *Gene Therapy for Hair Regrowth*. International Journal of Trichology, 9(4), 132–138.

53. Truong, C. Q., & Tran, P. (2016). *Advances in Hair Transplantation Technology.* Aesthetic Surgery Journal, 36(4), 476–484.

54. Vanderveken, F., & Jouret, G. (2019). *Exosomes in Hair Restoration Therapy.* Dermatologic Surgery, 45(1), 90–95.

55. Wang, X., & Sun, L. (2018). *Antioxidants in the Management of Hair Disorders.* Journal of Dermatological Science, 90(1), 1–9.

56. Yazdabadi, A., Whiting, D., & Rufaut, N. (2017). *Platelet-Rich Plasma for the Treatment of Androgenetic Alopecia: A Review of the Evidence.* Journal of Cutaneous Medicine and Surgery, 21(3), 233–239.

57. Zhang, Z., & Yang, C. (2017). *Effects of Hormonal Modulation in Androgenetic Alopecia.* Journal of Clinical Endocrinology and Metabolism, 102(4), 1394–1401.

58. Zhou, L., & Li, F. (2016). The Role of Gut Health in Hair Loss: The Gut-Hair Axis. Gut, 65(4), 610–621.

59. Zhu, Y., & Hu, H. (2017). *Melatonin in the Regulation of Hair Follicle Cycle and Growth.* Experimental Dermatology, 26(5), 341–345.

60. Zito, P. M., & Ross, J. S. (2021). *Trichology: A Critical Overview.* Dermatologic Clinics, 39(1), 23–29.

www.ingramcontent.com/pod-product-compliance
Lightning Source LLC
Chambersburg PA
CBHW071238020426
42333CB00015B/1522